D1125977

JOINT PAIN

By the Same Author

BACK PAIN

JOINT PAIN

Diagnosis and Treatment

Using Manipulative Techniques

by

John McM. Mennell, M.D.

Associate Professor, Department of Physical Medicine
and Rehabilitation, University of Pennsylvania School
of Medicine; Associate Professor, Department of Physical Medicine and Rehabilitation, Division of Graduate
Medicine, University of Pennsylvania School of Medicine; Attending Physician, Veterans Administration
Hospital, Philadelphia; Attending-Consultant, Bryn
Mawr Hospital, Bryn Mawr

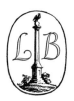

LITTLE, BROWN AND COMPANY

Boston

COPYRIGHT © 1964 BY JOHN MC M. MENNELL

ALL RIGHTS RESERVED. NO PART OF THIS BOOK MAY BE REPRO-
DUCED IN ANY FORM WITHOUT PERMISSION IN WRITING FROM THE
PUBLISHER, EXCEPT BY A REVIEWER WHO MAY QUOTE BRIEF PAS-
SAGES IN A REVIEW TO BE PRINTED IN A MAGAZINE OR NEWSPAPER

LIBRARY OF CONGRESS CATALOG CARD NO. 64-14259

FIRST EDITION

ISBN 0-316-56668

Fourth Printing

*Published in Great Britain
by Churchill/Livingstone, Edinburgh and London*

PRINTED IN THE UNITED STATES OF AMERICA

Preface

No technical book in the field of orthopedics can be entirely original. My object in this book is to summarize the experience of many years of practice and to present a detailed method of examining synovial joints by which may be elicited signs of a very common cause of joint pain — namely, *joint dysfunction* — that is largely unrecognized in clinical practice.

I hope this book will provide an increasing clinical appreciation of one more etiological factor that commonly causes pain in joints and will add to our knowledge of a ready way of relieving the symptoms of joint pain.

Although the use of manipulative techniques is controversial, their therapeutic value has been proved to my satisfaction. I trust that this work may help to establish my point and to advance the benefits of manipulative techniques which are, I believe, too often ignored in diagnosis and treatment.

It is extremely difficult to indicate movement in a static photograph. In the illustrations I have tried where technically practical to indicate movement more clearly by the use of double-exposure techniques. Arrows have been superimposed on the pictures to indicate the direction of pushes and pulls in the performance of the various movements being illustrated. When it has been possible to do so, wedges indicate the pivot points.

The number of x-ray illustrations to show what happens to

the joints, at least at the completion of the movements described, are limited, mainly by consideration of the possible ill effects to volunteer models of repeated exposure to irradiation.

The people to whom I am indebted in the production of this book are many indeed. Each knows his or her contribution and will, I trust, accept anonymously my thanks and my apology for failing to give specifically by name credit where credit is due.

My friend Fred Belliveau, Manager of the Medical Book Department of Little, Brown and Company, deserves all the credit for its conception and eventual publication. The patience he exhibited throughout is rare, and I am deeply grateful for it.

Tim Dodge and Ricardo Lopez of Long Beach Veterans Administration Hospital and Edward Gilfort of Philadelphia are responsible for the photographs. Without their remarkable skills the text would be of little value. Mrs. Elizabeth Braum of Long Beach Veterans Administration Hospital and Roger Shannon, M.D., prepared the line drawings, whose excellence needs no comment from me. My models were willing friends who wanted to help, and to all these people I extend profound thanks.

Almost a dozen of the illustrations and the text associated with them are taken from my book *Back Pain*. For the publisher's permission to use this material I am grateful. The greatest number of illustrations are official photographs of the Veterans Administration. I am grateful for permission to reproduce them.

Finally, I thank Mary C. Knox, my secretary, who labored uncomplainingly through so many extra hours of taxing work.

The motivation for all our efforts is the hope of having a medical book and its theories put successfully to clinical use in relieving patients who are in pain.

J. McM. M.

Seal Beach, California

Contents

JOINT PAIN

1

Preamble

There can be few physicians who, at one time or another, have not been baffled by the clinical fact that, after a joint has been immobilized for any reason, there is pain and stiffness in it. It is striking that the pain will disappear only after the stiffness has disappeared. This situation exists even in the absence of clinically or radiographically demonstrable signs of pathological changes within the joint. There are more times than there should be when such stiffness and pain persist; then, all too often, many of us try to explain it away by telling the patient, in a rather nebulous way, that the symptoms are due to "arthritis," an unavoidable complication.

Consideration of Normal Joint Movement

It is well known that loss of function in one joint may have widespread effects on the normal functioning of much of the rest of the musculoskeletal system; for example, it is the rare patient with disease of a hip who does not suffer from some back pain. Many a late-developing symptom of musculoskeletal pain could be easily avoided if one knew better how to care for current joint problems.

The causes of pain in synovial joints actually remain a mystery

1

to us. There are certain pathological conditions of joints that are commonly accepted as causing pain, but there is often no satisfactory explanation as to why and from where the pain arises in these conditions.

Joint Dysfunction

The contribution that I have to make is the recognition of one additional pathological condition which is readily reversible in its early stages and which, unlike the other well-recognized causes of pain, is common in life but cannot be demonstrated after death. For this very reason, it is difficult for those who rely on seeing pathological specimens in pathology lectures and museums to accept the condition as a pathological entity, which is not only diagnosable, but eminently treatable.

This condition I call *joint dysfunction;* it signifies a loss of joint-play movement that cannot be produced by the action of voluntary muscles, in contradistinction to the loss of a voluntary action of a joint which, together with pain, results from this condition. Having recognized joint dysfunction as a pain-producing pathological condition that causes loss of movement, I intend to show that restoration of normal joint play by manipulation is the logical and the only reasonable treatment to relieve pain from it and to restore normal voluntary movement.

Diagnosis. The recognition of dysfunction can only be achieved by clinical means. It is not demonstrable by routine static x-ray examination. The completion of any movement of joint play can be demonstrated by stress x-rays, which is demonstrated in some of the illustrations that follow. Stress x-rays, however, cannot be made routinely, if only because of the potential danger from repeated exposure to radiation of the operator's hands. Dysfunction also does not cause any biochemical alterations that may be detected by laboratory methods.

The detection of joint dysfunction, then, depends upon a method of clinical examination based on one's anatomical knowledge of the full range of movement that is normal to each individual synovial joint. There may be individual variations in the degree of joint play at any specific synovial joint, but there is no variation of technique in eliciting each movement at each joint. All normal movements of joint play are performed painlessly. If pain is elicited during the performance of a joint-play movement, this suggests that the movement is impaired. The degree of impairment can usually be determined by comparing the movement with that of the same joint on the other side of the body, which, fortunately in our work, is seldom involved.

Normal Joint Play

The normal range of joint movement taught in anatomy classes is that movement that is available to a normal joint produced by normal muscle action. These voluntary movements can be reproduced crudely in a cadaver, but they are the movements of dead anatomy.

In life, these voluntary movements cannot be achieved unless certain well-defined movements of joint play are present. Movements of joint play are independent of the action of the voluntary muscles. These joint-play movements are all very small but precise in range; it is upon their integrity that the easy, painless performance of movements in the voluntary range depends. Their integrity, not their range, is the basis of their importance. It is the summation of the movements of joint play and the movements in the voluntary range that make up the movements of living anatomy.

For the most part, then, this book must be recognized as a textbook of examining techniques. The actual movements of joint play which are normal to each joint and the method used to elicit them in normal joints are detailed in the appropriate topographical chapters. It is only by knowing what should be present in the way of movement in a normal joint that it is possible to detect its loss and, when appropriate, to know how to restore that which is lost.

In clinical teaching concerning problems of the musculoskeletal system, emphasis for the most part is placed on the deficiencies of the muscles in loss of function. As a result, treatment of these problems is usually directed at retraining and redeveloping the muscles — this, in spite of the fact that most of us know that loss of primary muscle function is confined to muscle diseases, myopathies, dystrophies, and neurological diseases. These conditions are relatively rare and are seldom accompanied by primary joint changes.

Commonly, joint disease is the cause of secondary muscle changes, particularly atrophy and spasm, the latter being protective and Nature's attempt reflexly to prevent painful joint movement. Yet, sparse attention is given in treatment to the joint itself unless there are gross clinical and radiographic changes in it, in which case treatment is often directed solely at the joint, and no attention is paid to the muscles.

This leads to reiteration of the basic truisms, which are too often neglected in practice, that: (1) when a joint is not free to move, the muscles that move it cannot be free to move it, (2) muscles cannot be restored to normal if the joints which they move are not free to move, (3) normal muscle function is dependent on normal joint movement, and (4) impaired muscle function perpetuates and may cause deterioration in abnormal joints.

There can be no doubt that there is a vicious circle of effects in any musculoskeletal problem, but, usually, the prime fault lies in the synovial joint. It is the detection of the prime fault in the synovial joints with which this present work is concerned. If the prime fault can be corrected, the secondary abnormalities resulting from it can usually be readily corrected, too.

Anatomy of Normal Joints

Basically, in any pure joint problem one is dealing with two bones, with their periosteal covering, the ends of which are covered with hyaline cartilage upon which the bone ends move. These articular surfaces are enclosed in a synovial capsule, which maintains sufficient synovial fluid for mechanical lubrication of the articular surfaces. The capsule is reinforced by well-defined ligaments that strengthen it to withstand stresses of use — or misuse.

In many joints, stability is maintained by the ligaments. In other joints, stabilization is achieved largely by muscle function. In still other joints, stability is achieved partially by the ligaments and partially by the muscles. For instance, the ankle joint is, for the most part, stabilized by ligaments; the shoulder joint mainly by muscles; and the knee joint by a combination of ligaments and muscles. In five joints of the body there are intra-articular fibrocartilages. And in certain well-defined anatomical locations there are bursae. There are thus seven anatomical structures that make up the synovial joints of the limbs, excluding the blood vessels, nerves and investing fascia and skin.

Differential Diagnosis of Joint Pain

The etiological conditions that may effect pathological changes in these anatomical structures are trauma, inflammation, metabolic disease, neoplasms, and congenital anomalies. Not all the pathological processes affect all the anatomical structures; so there are therefore less than thirty-five possible diagnoses in which pain arising from a joint is a symptom. But pain can only arise from a structure in which there is a sensory nerve supply or a vascular supply, the loss of which may produce ischemia with pain resulting. Hyaline cartilage and the intra-articular fibrocartilages are endowed with neither.

With this basic knowledge, there are three other clinical facts that assist in arriving at a diagnosis: first, synovial fluid is clinically unappreciable in a normal synovial joint; second, the synovial capsule cannot be palpated in its healthy state; and third, ligaments are tender only when they are torn or ruptured or when there is disease in the joint which they support.

Let us then consider the possible differential diagnoses of pain local to and arising from the shoulder — or glenohumeral joint. This joint is chosen because apparently it is a very simple joint and frequently the site of pain. Actually, it is a very complicated joint and illustrates particularly well the importance of joint play in the maintenance of joint function.

The local causes of shoulder pain are as follows: (1) fracture of one of the bones in relation to the joint, (2) dislocation of the joint, (3) traumatic synovitis of the joint, (4) traumatic hemarthrosis of the joint, (5) supraspinatus tendinitis (peritendinitis calcarea), (6) bicipital tendinitis, (7) rupture of the long head of the biceps, (8) a tear in the rotator cuff, (9) fibrositis in any of the large mobilizing muscles of the joint, (10) capsulitis (periarthritis), (11) osteochondritis, (12) osteomyelitis of any bone in relation to the joint, (13) neoplasm in any structure making up the joint, (14) pyarthrosis, (15) metabolic disease affecting any bone in relation to the joint, (16) "osteoarthritis," (17) bursitis — primary bursitis is rare, secondary bursitis is common

— and (18) *dysfunction* which may be primary but is residual from every other cause of pain in the shoulder and therefore the most common cause of pain.

Pain is commonly referred to one or the other shoulder joint from diseased viscera in the chest and in the upper abdomen, and from pathological conditions in the neck, cervical spine, axilla, and chest wall. Differential diagnosis of shoulder pain is sometimes especially difficult because any pain which is appreciated in the shoulder will affect the joint as though it were arising in it. Systemic disease may also present itself clinically as shoulder pain; collagen vascular diseases, gout, brucellosis, and some venereal diseases are examples.

The clue to the fact that the glenohumeral joint is far from simple (as anatomists would have us believe) is found in the shape of the glenoid process of the scapula. Far from being round or oval, it is pear-shaped, the large part of the pear being dependent.

At rest the head of the humerus articulates with the upper, smaller part of the glenoid cavity. In all useful voluntary function the head of the humerus articulates with the lower, larger part of the glenoid cavity. That the head of the humerus does glide downward and backward within the glenoid cavity during movement can be readily demonstrated radiographically and is easily appreciated clinically. If the reader places the tip of his forefinger over the superior aspect of another subject's greater tuberosity and then passively abducts the subject's arm from his side, at an early angle of abduction — less than 45 degrees — the tuberosity will suddenly disappear from beneath the palpating finger. This is because the head of the humerus has dropped downward into the large, dependent part of the glenoid cavity. If this movement is now repeated but with the index finger placed upon the anterior aspect of the greater tuberosity and the arm then forward flexed passively, again the tuberosity will, at an early angle of forward flexion, disappear from beneath the palpating finger. This is because the head of the humerus has glided backward within the glenoid cavity. Incidentally, these movements of gliding downward and backward of the head of the humerus within the glenoid cavity allow the greater tuberosity to slide beneath the acromion process. Were this not the case, the tuberosity would impinge upon the acromion process and pinch whatever soft tissue lies between the two bones. This soft tissue, of course, includes the subacromial bursa.

It is impossible by the use of the voluntary muscles to move the head of the humerus downward and backward within the glenoid cavity without raising the arm from the body in one way or another. These movements, therefore, are essentially involuntary and fall into that range of movement upon whose integrity the performance of voluntary movements depends. This, and a similar range of movement in all synovial joints, is *the range of movement of joint play*.

If, for any reason, pain is felt in a shoulder, whether it is caused by a local pathological condition in the shoulder joint or by some distant pathological process from which pain is referred to the shoulder joint, the muscles of the shoulder respond, as muscles do in any location to the stimulus of pain, by going into spasm. This spasm occurs with the shoulder in the position of rest, and if unrelieved, it holds the head of the humerus so that it articulates with the upper, useless part of the glenoid cavity. In this situation, when voluntary movement is attempted, the head of the humerus can no longer glide downward and backward within the glenoid cavity because the movements of joint play are lost, and very quickly a frozen shoulder results.

The loss of these movements of joint play may be primary, in which case it is usually the result of minor trauma, often caused by some unguarded, and therefore abnormal, movement of the joint being inflicted upon the joint during the performance of an otherwise normal voluntary movement. In this case, the loss of joint play, that is, dysfunction, is a diagnosis of the cause of pain and limitation of voluntary movement. In a case of primary dysfunction the treatment to relieve the pain and loss of function is to restore those movements of joint play that have been lost. This is the *treatment of manipulation.*

Dysfunction — A Diagnosis or a Clinical Sign

Dysfunction, however, is also an invaluable sign of some serious pathological process or joint disease. The differentiation of dysfunction the diagnosis and dysfunction the sign of disease can only be made by meticulous examination, which includes history taking, clinical examination, radiographic study, and often laboratory investigation.

When dysfunction is a sign of more serious joint disease, it will remain, even after the primary disease is eradicated, and will then become a primary cause of residual pain in the joint which can only be readily relieved by manipulation. It should be obvious, however, that manipulative treatment for dysfunction is courting disaster if it is used before any primary active disease process is eradicated.

Unfortunately, about the only way to determine the time at which dysfunction, the sign of disease, becomes dysfunction, the primary cause of residual symptoms following the eradication of the disease, is clinical experience. However, there is one historical feature which strongly suggests that this has occurred and that is that the patient will volunteer that the nature of his symptoms has changed and that, whereas, during the stage of the active inflammation his symptoms were worse and that the

joint became stiffer after rest, his symptoms are now improved
by rest. At this point gentle but firm manipulative examination
will not cause an exacerbation of his symptoms in the 24 hours
following their application, whereas, during the active inflammatory phase, even the gentlest examining maneuvers produced
an exacerbation of symptoms, lasting maybe up to 24 hours.

The gliding downward and backward of the head of the
humerus on the glenoid cavity are but two of the seven movements of joint play upon whose integrity the voluntary function
of the shoulder joint depends. The full range of joint-play movement is described in the topographical chapter concerning the
shoulder joint (Chap. 8, page 78).

The movements of joint play in the various joints of the extremities described in the later topographical chapters are simply
the normal involuntary movements that are present at each normal synovial joint and that must be present before the voluntary
muscles can move the joint through its normal voluntary range
of movement. These movements in this context have nothing to
do with manipulative treatment. Certainly, they are manipulative movements, but they are movements of examination and
must not be confused with those therapeutic maneuvers that are
used to restore these movements when they are lost, that is, when
the cause of joint pain and limitation of voluntary joint movement results from dysfunction. That the manipulative therapeutic
maneuvers are, in most cases, identical with the examining
maneuvers, must not cloud the issue that the topographical chapters describe what is normal anatomically and physiologically
in the joints for which they are described.

Joint Manipulation — A Therapy

It has always seemed to me that the main reason why the
medical profession has been reluctant to accept manipulative

therapy in the treatment of joint pain is because the proponents of manipulative treatment have never clearly emphasized that manipulative maneuvers in treatment are designed solely to restore something which is normal anatomically and physiologically to a joint — something which is unconcerned with voluntary joint movement but is solely concerned with mechanical joint play, and which is essentially present only in life and absent in death. The prerequisite for successful treatment in any field of medicine is accurate diagnosis. The condition of joint dysfunction is the only pathological condition that will respond to the treatment of manipulation. So, before manipulative therapy is ever used, the normal range of joint-play movements must be learned as carefully as the range of voluntary movement is now taught and learned in routine anatomy classes. That joint-play movements are small, often not more than $\frac{1}{8}$ of an inch in extent in any plane, does not mean that they are unimportant. It is, in fact, upon the integrity of these small, precise, involuntary movements that the performance of the gross voluntary movements of synovial joints depends.

2

History Taking

Causes of Joint Pain

The importance of taking a meticulous history cannot be too highly emphasized if diagnostic errors are to be avoided. It is stressed again, however, that this work is primarily concerned with the diagnosis and treatment of joint dysfunction which, by definition, signifies the loss of one or more movements in the normal range of joint play, and this loss of movement is the cause of pain. Joint dysfunction is merely one possible diagnosis, and it must be differentiated from the many other causes of joint pain. Just as there are many clues in a patient's history of joint pain which may point to the diagnosis of joint disease, so also are there clues available from a patient's history which strongly suggest the diagnosis of joint dysfunction. There is little new, therefore, in the following paragraphs on history taking from a patient complaining of joint pain, but some of the interpretations of the various points in the history may be found to have new significance.

Etiological Factors Predisposing to Joint Dysfunction. Primary joint dysfunction commonly results from the imposition of some unguarded movement at a joint that at the time is actively going through a normal functional movement. It may also com-

12

monly follow some definite traumatic episode of a minor nature involving the joint, the immediate effects of which are usually diagnosed as sprains or strains. In the former case, the trauma to the joint is intrinsic whereas in the latter case it is extrinsic. The recognition that a joint can be injured from an intrinsic cause is essential to the appreciation of the condition of joint dysfunction.

Joint dysfunction is perhaps the commonest cause of residual symptoms after severe bone and joint injury and after almost every joint disease when the primary pathological condition has been eradicated, has healed, or is quiescent. Joint dysfunction commonly occurs in joints that have been immobilized in the treatment of fractures, even though there may be no particular reason to believe that the joints themselves were involved in the traumatic incident that caused the fractures. It may also follow immobilization occasioned either by severe soft tissue injury around the joint or by treatment following surgery. It is also the commonest cause of residual symptoms following any inflammatory condition of a joint or following the resolution of any systemic disease that involves joint structures. It may or may not be associated with the presence of intra-articular adhesions.

Present Complaint

Onset of Symptoms. The history of the onset of the joint symptoms may suggest a diagnosis. When dealing with joint problems the onset of symptoms is either sudden or insidious. If the onset is sudden and follows a remembered traumatic episode, but without associated joint swelling, joint dysfunction is a likely diagnosis. If the onset is sudden and the pain is accompanied by swelling of the joint, it is unlikely that joint dysfunction is the primary cause of the patient's symptoms; it is more probable that the symptoms are due to some pathological change in one or more of the seven anatomical structures that make up the joint. If the onset of symptoms is sudden, following, for instance, the removal of some supporting device that has been worn for any length of time, and coinciding with the resumption of activity, then it is most likely that the cause of pain is joint dysfunction.

If the onset of symptoms is insidious, joint dysfunction is a most unlikely diagnosis. It should be remembered, however, that intrinsic trauma to a joint may occur during sleep without wakening the patient, and the patient may only notice the discomfort or pain on waking. In such cases, when trauma is not recalled and the onset is considered to be insidious, the history must not be allowed to confuse the issue.

If more than one joint is involved and the onset of pain occurred at about the same time, joint dysfunction can be the cause only if the involved joints have been immobilized as part of treatment, for example, after multiple fractures, burns, or a single fracture in which the immobilizing cast extends over more than one joint, or if there is a very clear history of a traumatic episode that definitely involves all the joints in which there is pain.

Nature of Joint Pain. The pain of joint dysfunction tends to be sharp and occurs, often only intermittently, when the joint is in function, the same movement always causing recurrence of the pain. It is almost always relieved by rest.

When joint dysfunction causes residual symptoms after a primary joint disease or injury has been eradicated or become quiescent, the history of the nature of the pain changes. It is this change in the nature of the pain that gives the clue that the residual symptoms in the joint are probably arising from joint dysfunction. During the phase of active disease, for example, the patient finds that the pain is possibly worse after rest and that the joint stiffens with rest, whereas with joint dysfunction the patient finds the pain is improved by rest and is disturbing only when the joint is used.

Joint pain that is disturbing to the patient on waking in the morning, is less severe after he limbers up with perhaps an hour or more of activity, and then worsens again toward the end of the day, is seldom due to joint dysfunction. Night pain that wakens the patient is often due to bone disease or neoplasm.

The pain of joint disease is most often deep, aching, and throbbing; it may be lessened by pressure just as the ache from an infected tooth may be somewhat relieved by pressing on it. This type of pain may be constant or occur in waves or spasms, and it may be sharp or dull. The pain of joint dysfunction is invariably sharp; it usually ceases immediately when the stressful action that produces it ceases; it is invariably relieved or at least markedly improved by rest and aggravated by activity. Thus the patient's answers to questions as to what aggravates and what improves the pain may be very significant.

Localization of Pain. The localization of the pain by the patient is sometimes most helpful in giving a clue to a correct diagnosis, for often patients are able to indicate clearly in which component of the joint the pain seems to be situated when the pathological condition causing the pain is not joint dysfunction. In the areas of the limbs where there are multiple joints, the localization of the pain by the patient will often draw attention to the specific joint from which the pain is arising and in which dysfunction may be present.

Loss of Movement and Pain. In the joints of the limbs, each movement in the range of joint play is always associated with the ability to perform some particular voluntary motion. For instance, extension at the wrist for the most part occurs at the midcarpal joint. If a patient is unable to extend the wrist, this fact should draw attention to the movements of joint play upon which the voluntary movement of extension depends, namely, those which are associated with the midcarpal joint. In the same region, inability of the patient to perform supination of the forearm following, for example, a Colles' fracture should draw attention to the joint-play movements associated with either the ulnomeniscotriquetral joint or the inferior radioulnar joint, or both.

Past History

The past history of a patient complaining of joint pain must be inquired into for therein may lie the clue to the true nature of the pathological cause of the pain. A past history of heart disease in childhood, chorea, or St. Vitus dance suggests that the cause of pain may be acute rheumatic fever. Migraine or allergic conditions such as asthma or hay fever suggest a diagnosis of nonspecific intermittent hydrarthrosis. A chronic cough, loss of weight, unexplained pyrexia, undue sweating, and the drinking of raw milk in the past suggest that the underlying cause of the joint symptoms may be tuberculosis or brucellosis, whereas fleeting pains in the small joints of the extremities are suggestive of rheumatoid arthritis. Joint pain following dietary extravagance may suggest gout, and the history of a recent injection of antitoxin or the administration of a new drug might suggest an allergic basis for the joint symptoms. Recent venereal disease may mean gonococcal arthritis, and syphilis may be manifested in either synovial or bony changes in a joint. The history of recent intra-articular injections of medication or of joint aspiration may suggest the onset of pyarthrosis. In the joints in which there are intra-articular fibrocartilages (menisci), a past history of locking of the joint with pain strongly suggests meniscal injury.

The past history may reveal illness while traveling abroad, and it should be remembered that hydatid disease, amebiasis, fungal infections, and some rare tropical diseases may manifest themselves as joint pain in their chronic course.

Family History

The patient's family history should not be forgotten, for there is a tendency for rheumatic diseases to be familial. This work, however, is not concerned with the more esoteric causes of joint pain such as ochronosis and hemophilia from which the differentiation of joint dysfunction should present no problem.

System Review

A complete review of a patient's visceral systems should be undertaken since joint pain may be the presenting feature of systemic disease such as lupus erythematosus, scleroderma, dermatomyositis, Reiter's disease, erythema nodosum, and polyarteritis nodosa. Symptoms of joint pain may rarely be associated with and draw attention to acromegaly, pulmonary disease, kidney disease, and Henoch's purpura and other hemorrhagic dyscrasias. Arthralgia may also be associated with ulcerative colitis.

Pain in a joint may be referred from disease of a distant viscera which may be diagnosed only by careful system review. Classic examples of this fact include a wide variety of conditions often causing referred pain in a shoulder joint. A few of these are coronary artery disease, pericarditis, lesions in other parts of the mediastinum, empyema, pneumothorax, Pancoast's tumor, gall-bladder disease, peptic ulcer, diaphragmatic hernia, subphrenic abscess, and perisplenitis. Causalgic pain must be differentiated from somatic pain when involvement of the autonomic nervous system may be the cause of the symptoms. The recognition of a neuropathic joint which, contrary to the usual teaching, is by no means necessarily painless, may lead to the diagnosis of a disease such as syringomyelia, neurosyphilis, or diabetes.

Finally, although joint pain may be arising primarily from joint dysfunction, the pain in the joint may persist in spite of adequate treatment because of a secondary low-grade infective arthritis arising from some distant focus of infection such as teeth, tonsils, sinuses, and the genitourinary and gastrointestinal tracts, symptoms of which may be revealed during discussion of the patient's system review.

Differential Diagnostic Clues from Observation

There are certain interesting and peculiar features that on clinical observation may suggest the correct diagnosis of joint pain. For instance, pain which migrates from joint to joint in a patient who shows clinical evidence of systemic illness is very suggestive of rheumatic fever. The single painful joint that is apparently so painful that the patient withdraws it as the examiner prepares to examine it is very suggestive of the acute gonococcal joint. What appears to be a relatively mild problem in a single joint, but with more marked associated muscle atrophy than expected, is often the tuberculous joint. In considering the joints of the fingers, it is often said that osteoarthritis affects the distal interphalangeal joints, that rheumatoid arthritis affects the proximal interphalangeal joints, and that gout affects the metacarpophalangeal joints. Joint pain from gout is by no means limited to the feet, nor is it by any means always associated with tophi; gout may occur in any of the joints of the limbs and even in the joints of the vertebral column. The less common forms of arthritis may be suggested to the diagnostician only by the absence of the diagnostic features of the more common causes of joint pain.

The relationship of osteoarthritis to the diagnosis and treatment of joint pain is very cogent to this thesis but is dealt with in a later chapter (Chap. 16, page 154). It is sufficient to say here that I do not believe that osteoarthritis per se causes pain in joints. It is my belief that the commonest cause of pain in an osteoarthritic joint is joint dysfunction.

Traumatic Synovitis and Hemarthrosis

The other important problem at this time, and one which is too often neglected by the physician, is the clinical differentiation of traumatic synovitis from hemarthrosis. The correct, early treatment of these conditions may well save a patient from disabling residual joint pain and from pathological changes which develop many years later. By definition, the onset of both of these conditions follows trauma to a joint. Both conditions are associated with articular swelling; however, the swelling of hemarthrosis is rapid and follows the trauma immediately, whereas the swelling of traumatic synovitis is slow and may not occur for twenty-four hours. The size of the swelling in hemarthrosis is small, whereas the size of the swelling in synovitis is often quite great. The joint which contains blood is a hot and acutely painful joint, whereas the joint in which the swelling is due to excess synovial fluid is usually warm and aching.

The importance of differentiating these two conditions clinically is that fluid should not be withdrawn from a joint in which there is simple synovitis, whereas the removal of blood from a joint at the earliest possible moment is mandatory. The reason that I believe that the joint with simple traumatic synovitis should not be aspirated is that synovial fluid is normal to the joint, and excess fluid will be absorbed normally as soon as the pathological condition that has given rise to its excess has resolved. Its presence in excess, therefore, is the best clinical indication that all is not well within the joint; if it does not disappear spontaneously, then either the diagnosis is wrong or the treatment is wrong, or both. Also, the unnecessary introduction of a needle into a joint should be avoided because of the chances of introducing infection.

The excess synovial fluid of traumatic synovitis will, of course, never disappear so long as the joint is subjected to the repetitive minor trauma of use while the active traumatic injury is present. Thus, the correct treatment of traumatic synovitis is rest from function, but not rest from movement; however, the movement part of the treatment must never cause pain. This is probably the most important teaching in the treatment of any joint problem, for if this movement concept were followed more assiduously in the treatment of joints afflicted by various pathological conditions, there would be far fewer disabling residues from joint injury. However, it must be made perfectly clear that movement in this context may mean simply one or two degrees of movement, and by no means denotes putting the joint through anything resembling its normal range of voluntary movement.

Clues Suggesting Joint Dysfunction

In review, when joint dysfunction is the primary cause of joint pain, the clues in the patient's history are that the symptom of pain was sudden in onset, occurred following some unguarded joint movement, was unassociated with marked swelling or warmth, is limited to one joint, and that the pain is lessened by rest, which does not produce stiffness, and is aggravated by activity.

3

Examination—
General Considerations

The examination techniques described in the following topographical chapters are certainly not meant to replace the routine methods used in the clinical examination of synovial joints. They are additional examination techniques to be used to determine the presence of impairment of the normal movements of joint play, or their absence, in the joint being examined.

Again, it must be stressed that adequate history taking may be the most important part of the clinical investigation of a patient complaining of joint pain. Any abbreviation of this must result in errors in diagnosis.

General Physical Examination

Temperature and Pulse. The patient's temperature and pulse should be noted before any examination of a painful joint is undertaken. This may be a trite observation, but these two simple examining procedures are too often overlooked.

Inspection. Any painful joint should be inspected before it is palpated or moved. The color of the skin and the presence or absence of swelling should be noted. The alteration of muscle contour or noticeable muscle atrophy is important. The appearance of the contralateral, normal limb should always be compared to that of the limb in which the affected joint is situated.

Palpation. Before the joint is moved at all, it should be palpated at rest. At this time differences of local skin temperature, the presence of fluctuation within the joint, the consistency of the synovial capsule and the consistency of the supporting and mobilizing muscles of the joint must be noted. If, for instance, on examining a knee joint that by history is limited in movement and is painful following the healing of a fracture of one of the bones of the leg, and if there is obvious fibrosis and binding down of the quadriceps expansion which invariably is associated with atrophy of the quadriceps, it should be immediately obvious that the patella is fixed in its cephalad range of movement. In this position, the patella blocks flexion of the knee, and it is impossible to restore movement to the knee joint until the patella is mobilized. Nor, in these circumstances, can it be anticipated that normal physiology can be restored to the quadriceps muscle until the fibrotic changes in the quadriceps expansion are reversed. The prescription of mobilizing procedures to the joint or an exercise program for the muscle must fail.

The ligaments of the joint being examined must all be palpated individually because it is classic that ligaments are never tender unless they are torn or ruptured, or there is some pathological condition within the joint which they support. It should also be remembered that the normal capsule of a joint cannot be appreciated by palpation. If the capsule can be palpated, then there is either some pathological condition within the joint or in the synovium itself.

Examination of Movements in the Voluntary Range. In the presence of signs of active inflammation within the joint, which can be detected by the examination procedures described up to this point, it is then unnecessary to examine joint movement at all. Examination of joint movement in infants under these conditions may indeed be disastrous.

In the absence of signs of active inflammation within the joint, movement of the joint in its voluntary range should be noted as it is performed actively by the patient and then should be checked by passive examination. The degrees of movement in each normal range of movement should be noted as a baseline from which improvement or deterioration can be checked and also for comparison with the unaffected side. When the pain is in a joint of one of the lower extremities, any inequality of leg length should be noted, since this may cause unnatural stresses of weight bearing at otherwise normal joints and may result in joint dysfunction from relatively innocuous unguarded movements. It also may result in early changes of traumatic osteoarthritis, or it may cause laxity of the supporting ligaments from constant repetitive strain from otherwise normal function. Any insufficiency of the Achilles tendons should be noted; the importance of Achilles tendon insufficiency is discussed in some detail in Chapter 16, pages 161–165.

Study of the gait may prove an important aid in diagnosis. A gluteus medius gait is commonly associated with pathological changes in the hip joint, for instance. It should be remembered that the examination of a painful knee joint is incomplete until the hip joint on the same side has been examined also. Any child complaining of pain in the knee has a pathological condition in the hip of the same side until it is proved that he does not.

Muscle Examination. The mobilizing and stabilizing muscles of the involved joint must then be examined. Muscle atrophy may be appreciated by inspection, but it can also be checked quite accurately in certain situations by measurements. In considering knee joint pain, it is particularly important to assess atrophy of the vastus medialis accurately. In the average patient, circumferential measurement of the thigh at 2 inches above the patella will detect masked synovial swelling in the suprapatellar pouch. Circumferential measurement of the thigh at 4 inches above the patella will specifically detect atrophy of the vastus medialis, which is invariably present with pathological conditions of the knee joint. Measurement of the circumference of the thigh more proximal to this point detects group muscle atrophy, which is more commonly associated with pathological conditions of the spine. As long as there is any atrophy or weakness of a vastus medialis a knee will remain unstable, even after the successful treatment and eradication of any pathological cause of pain within the knee joint. Since the vastus medialis comes into full play only in the last 15 degrees of voluntary extension of the knee joint, re-educative exercises prescribed for the quadriceps muscles often fail to restore normal strength and function to the vastus medialis because of the inadequate way a patient is taught to do the exercises. Too often the importance of the last 15 degrees of movement is not stressed so that the patient fails to concentrate on completing full extension.

Muscle weakness may occur without atrophy, though this is unlikely. A manual muscle test is often an important part of the clinical examination and provides another baseline from which improvement or deterioration of a pathological condition in the joint may be assessed. Electrical muscle tests are of value only when some interruption of the neuromuscular mechanism is suspected. Muscle volume and power should always be compared with that on the unaffected side.

X-ray Examination

The habit of looking at the x-ray films of a joint before the clinical examination is made must be deprecated. Obvious radiographic joint changes are too frequently blamed for symptoms, which results in their real cause's being overlooked. X-rays, for the most part, should be used to confirm a clinical diagnosis and not to make it. There are no characteristic radiographic changes in joints to suggest the diagnosis of joint dysfunction, and joint dysfunction may be present and giving rise to symptoms in the absence of any radiographic changes at all. On the other hand, radiographic changes characteristic of osteoarthritis, for example, may be present when the only cause of symptoms is joint dysfunction. A consultation between the radiologist and the examining clinician may be essential before one can determine the importance of the radiographic findings. A radiological report should be accepted only in conjunction with personal examination of the x-ray film.

Sometimes special x-ray techniques are needed before an accurate diagnosis of joint pathology can be arrived at. Stress radiographs may have to be taken to determine the integrity of the supporting ligaments of a joint. Stereoscopic films may help to determine the localization of loose bodies within the joint. Depth estimations may have to be made by the radiologist to determine whether foreign bodies are intra-articular or extra-articular. Some advocate the use of arthrograms, and certainly they may be useful diagnostically, especially in determining the presence of a tear in a joint capsule in which case a radiopaque dye is used. In some instances the presence of traumatic injury of an intra-articular fibrocartilage can be determined when air is used as the contrast medium.

Laboratory Procedures

Certain laboratory tests may be required before an accurate diagnosis of the cause of joint pain can be arrived at. A complete blood count and sedimentation rate should be almost routine. A determination of the serum uric acid may lead to the diagnosis of gout. An estimation of the albumin-globulin ratio and the performance of the usual complement fixation tests, flocculation tests, and agglutination tests may be necessary before conditions such as rheumatoid arthritis, brucellosis, typhoid fever, or syphilis, for instance, can be diagnosed or ruled out. A hematologic study for lupus erythematosus may be necessary, and such nonspecific determinations as the C-reactive protein may be useful in conjunction with other laboratory signs. Certainly, serial determinations of the antistreptolysin-O titer may be essential in revealing or following the activity of rheumatic fever. The heterophile antibody may reveal infectious mononucleosis to be the underlying problem. Sickle-cell disease in a Negro may give the clue to the correct diagnosis. Parasitic ova may have to be sought for in the stools. Urinalysis, urine culture, and such things as throat culture and blood cultures may have to be done. Skin tests may also be necessary.

A painful joint may have to be aspirated for diagnostic purposes. The cellular content of synovial fluid may give a clue to the pathological condition within the joint, and the synovial fluid may have to be cultured to determine the organism causing infection and its sensitivity to antibiotics. There are times when synovial biopsy is essential to arrive at a correct diagnosis of the cause of joint pain.

Examination for Movements of Joint Play

While it is true that many of the foregoing auxiliary diagnostic procedures are often unnecessary and even redundant in
arriving at the correct diagnosis of the cause of the pain in a
joint, they have been discussed in this order to re-emphasize the
fact that the thesis of this work is that joint dysfunction is but
an additional diagnostic conclusion to be arrived at in assessing
a problem of joint pain. By the same token, it should not be
forgotten that it is also pertinent to this thesis that joint dysfunction is one of the commonest causes of joint pain in clinical
medicine. Evidence of joint dysfunction is therefore sought
early, in the absence of any clinical signs to suggest more serious joint disease.

Rules for Joint-Play Examination. To examine for joint-
play movements, the patient must be recumbent; only in this
position does the examiner have perfect control of the examining movements that he is performing. The only exception to
this is the examination of the joints of the fingers and those at
the wrists. The position of examination is vital to the accumu-
lation of precise data relating to joint movement. The techniques of eliciting joint play must be adhered to. It must be
remembered that joint-play movements, for the most part, are
small in range, and therefore their performance requires accu-
racy and precision.

In addition, there are certain rules of examining technique
which must be followed when using manipulative maneuvers.

(1) The patient must be relaxed and each aspect of the joint
being examined must be supported and protected from unguarded painful movement which may otherwise occur in the
course of the examination. Unguarded movements of painful
joints produce pain which puts the supporting muscles into

spasm and prevents the performance of the examining movements for joint play.

(2) The examiner must be relaxed. At no time must his examining "grip" be painful to the patient. The grasp that he uses must be firm and protective, but not restrictive.

(3) One joint must be examined at a time. For instance, the wrist is not examined as such, but rather the radiocarpal joint, the midcarpal joint, the ulnomeniscocarpal joint and, finally, the inferior radioulnar joint are each examined in turn.

(4) One movement at each joint is examined at a time.

(5) In the performance of any one movement, one facet of the joint being examined is moved upon the other facet of the joint which is stabilized. Thus there should always be one mobilizing force and one stabilizing force exerted when a joint is being examined.

(6) The extent of normal joint play can usually be ascertained by examining the same joint in the unaffected limb.

(7) No forceful movement must ever be used, and no abnormal movement must ever be used.

(8) An examining movement must be stopped at any point at which pain is elicited. This is in contradistinction to Rule 8 in the rules concerning therapeutic techniques using manipulative maneuvers described in Chapter 14, page 135.

(9) In the presence of obvious clinical signs of joint (or bone) inflammation or disease, no examining movements need be or should be undertaken.

Exceptions to Rules of Joint-Play Examination. In the following chapters, which describe topographically the specific manipulation techniques used in the examination of painful joints when searching for evidence of joint dysfunction, it will be noted that Rules 3 and 4 above are frequently broken. For example, reference to Figures 19, 25, and 38 which follow will

show that the examining maneuver for eliciting long axis extension of the midcarpal joint, the radiocarpal joint, and the ulnomeniscotriquetral joint, as well as the maneuver for pulling the
head of the radius downward on the ulna, are all the same.
Later it will be noted in Figure 92B that the movement of long
axis extension at the midcarpal and radiocarpal joints is being
performed while the head of the humerus is being pulled downward in the glenoid cavity. Similarly, it will be noted when re-
ferring to Figures 62, 67, 69A, 69B, and then to Figures 71
and 72 that almost the identical manipulative maneuver is being
used for examination of long axis extension at the mortise joint
and the subtalar joint, and in performing the talar rock and the
lateral tilt movements of the calcaneous on the talus. In fact,
it will be noted that Figures 62 and 67 are identical, and the
photograph used to illustrate Figures 19, 25, and 38 is the same
in each case.

With regard to the examination of the joints of the upper
limbs, it is surprising how seldom both the midcarpal and the
radiocarpal joints are affected at the same time by joint dysfunction from any cause. In searching for impairment of the
long axis extension, at either joint, one is simply taking up the
slack of normal long axis extension of the uninvolved joint to
determine its presence or absence in the other joint. If dysfunction is present in both joints, then one is simply examining both
joints at the same time; no harm can come from this since the
same movement is being used and is normal for each joint. I
do not believe that I remember ever finding evidence of loss of
the joint-play movement of long axis extension at the ulnomeniscotriquetral joint, and this presumably is because the articulating surfaces of the two bones are separated relatively widely
by the intra-articular meniscus.

The downward movement of the head of the radius on the

ulna, which is accomplished by using the same technique, is legitimate if there is no involvement of the midcarpal or radio-carpal joints. The performance of these movements is simply part of taking up the slack before exerting the manipulative pull to move the head of the radius. If all three joints happen to be involved, again no harm can come from performing all three movements at one time since the pull for all is identical and normal. The same criteria hold for exerting the therapeutic manipulative maneuver of pulling the head of the humerus downward in the glenoid cavity at the maximum angle of arm abduction (see Chap. 15).

When we come to discuss long axis extension at the mortise joint and the subtalar joint in the lower extremity, the same rationalization must be allowed. It is strange clinically how often long axis extension is impaired at the subtalar joint without there being any impairment of the same movement at the mortise joint. However, in eliciting the joint-play movements of the talar rock and side tilt medially and laterally at the subtalar joint, Rules 3 and 4 are deliberately broken. But I do believe that these are the only times when this is so. The key word of the foregoing sentence is "deliberately." The only time that the user of manipulative techniques may break these rules is when he knowingly does it for a specific reason. If the rules are broken unknowingly, damage may be inflicted upon the joint being examined. If the rules are broken unknowingly when a thera-peutic manipulation is being performed, severe injury may be inflicted upon the joint being treated, and the novice will blame the procedure rather than his lack of knowledge of the tech-nique for the worsening of the joint condition and the failure of the treatment to bring his patient relief.

4

The Fingers

The Metacarpophalangeal and Interphalangeal Joints

The range of joint play in the metacarpophalangeal joints and in the interphalangeal joints is the same in movement but differs in extent. The metacarpophalangeal joint of the index finger is used to illustrate the techniques of examination of the range of joint-play movements in all these joints. The movements of joint play at this joint are: (1) long axis extension, (2) antero-posterior tilt, (3) side tilt medially and laterally, and (4) rotation. Also, because the metacarpophalangeal joint of the index finger is the most easily handled joint in the body and because it is a joint which is most readily and easily visualized radiographically, the joint-play movements at this joint are demonstrated radiographically to illustrate the extent of movement that is being achieved on examination. Reference to these radiographic illustrations will make it clear that the extent of the movements of joint play is small when compared to the extent of the voluntary movements which are dependent upon them. The fact that they are small does not mean that their importance is not great. Because the movements are small, however, it is of vital importance that they should be performed precisely.

Long Axis Extension. The examiner holds the head of the

metacarpal bone between his thumb and index finger and then grasps the shaft of the proximal phalanx as he would a golf club. He then pulls the base of the phalanx away from the head of the metacarpal bone. It should be noted clinically that, on

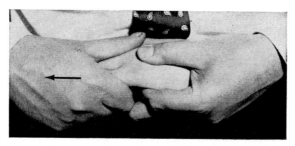

FIGURE 1. Long axis extension at a metacarpophalangeal joint, illustrating the golf-club grip by the examiner's mobilizing right hand and stabilization of the head of the metacarpal bone by his left hand. Arrow shows direction of pull by examiner.

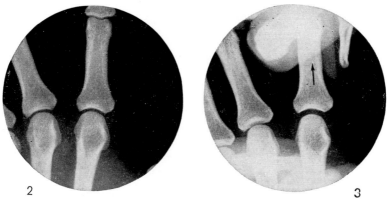

FIGURE 2. X-ray of the metacarpophalangeal joint of the index finger at rest.

FIGURE 3. X-ray of the metacarpophalangeal joint of the index finger at the limit of long axis extension. The relationship of the articulating surfaces of the bones should be compared with their relationship with the joint at rest (Figure 2). Arrow indicates direction of pull by examiner.

completion of long axis extension, none of the soft tissue structures are stretched; only the normal slack in them is taken up.

Figure 1 illustrates the position adopted to perform this joint-
play movement of long axis extension. Figure 2 demonstrates
radiographically the relationship of the same two bones prior
to the movement, that is, with the joint at rest, and Figure
3 demonstrates radiographically the relationship of the articular
surfaces of the bones at the end of the movement of long axis
extension. One should note the wide separation of the bones at
the completion of the movement of long axis extension (Figure
3), when compared to their relative positions at rest (Figure
2). The radial relationship of subchondral bone surfaces at rest
should also be noticed, since this relationship is maintained
throughout all the voluntary movements of this joint. For example, the relationship is maintained when the joint is flexed,

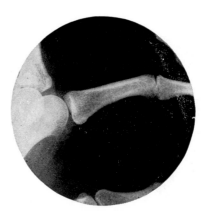

FIGURE 4. X-ray of the metacarpophalangeal joint of the index finger in flexion. Note that the radial
relationship of the articulating surfaces of the bones is the same as
that when the finger is at rest
(Figure 2).

as shown in Figure 4, whereas it differs widely in the performance of joint-play movements.

Anteroposterior Tilt. The examiner maintains his grip upon
the head of the metacarpal bone. He then places the tip of the
thumb of his other hand just distal to the base of the phalanx
posteriorly and the tip of his index finger just distal to the base
of the phalanx anteriorly. By applying pressure with the thumb
and the index finger alternately, he then tilts the base of the
phalanx alternately backward and forward, using either the
thumb or the index finger as a fulcrum. Thus the metacarpophalangeal joint is tilted open, first posteriorly and then anteriorly. To elicit these movements, the joint is held in about 10
degrees of flexion. Figure 5 shows the position adopted to elicit
these tilt movements.

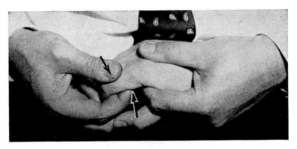

FIGURE 5.   The posterior tilt resulting from the posterior phase of
the anteroposterior tilt of the metacarpophalangeal joint of the index
finger. Note the examiner's right index finger is used as a pivot anteriorly, while the thumb presses toward the floor.

One should observe that these are not shearing movements
but pure tilting movements that open up the joint space anteriorly and posteriorly, again without stretching any of the supporting soft tissues. Figure 6 shows radiographically the rela-

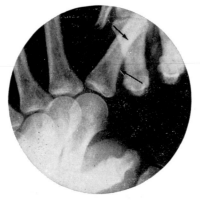

FIGURE 6. X-ray of the posterior tilt phase of the anteroposterior tilt of the metacarpophalangeal joint. The difference in the radial relationship of the articulating surfaces of the bones in this position and their relationship in flexion (Figure 4) should be noted.

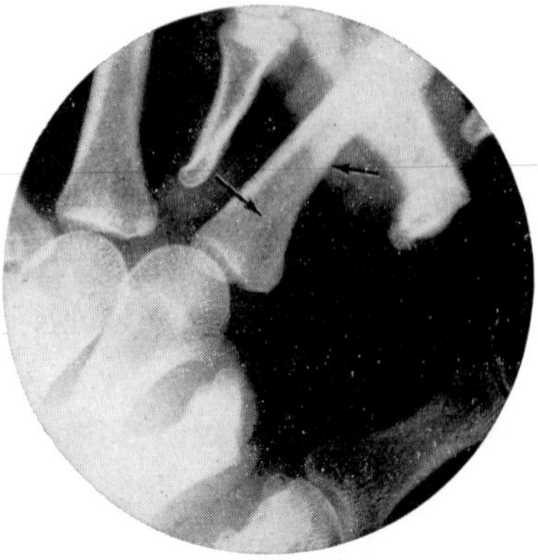

FIGURE 7. X-ray of the anterior tilt phase of the anteroposterior tilt of the metacarpophalangeal joint. The difference in the radial relationship of the articulating surfaces of the bones in this position and their relationship in flexion (Figure 4) should be noted.

tionship of the articular surfaces of the bones at the limit of the posterior phase of this movement, whereas Figure 7 shows their relationship at the limit of the anterior phase of this movement.

The position of the base of the phalanx in relation to the head of the metacarpal bone should be noted in the voluntary movements of flexion (see Figure 4) and be compared with their relative positions when the joint space is tilted open in the movements of joint play (see Figures 6 and 7).

Side Tilt. The examiner maintains his grip on the head of the metacarpal bone. He places the thumb and index finger of the other hand on the medial and lateral side of the proximal phalanx, respectively, just distal to its base. Using the thumb as a pivot, the metacarpophalangeal joint is tilted open medially by exerting pressure through the tip of the index finger. Then, using the tip of the index finger as a pivot, the metacarpophalangeal joint is tilted open laterally by exerting pressure through the

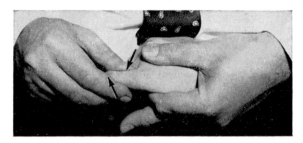

FIGURE 8.   Lateral tilt opening up the lateral aspect of a metacarpophalangeal joint. Note the examiner's right thumb is being used as a pivot, while his index finger tilts the base of the phalanx away from the metacarpal bone.

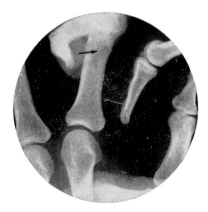 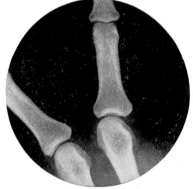

FIGURE 9.   X-ray of the side tilt of the metacarpophalangeal joint tilted open medially. The radial relationship of the articulating surfaces of the bones in this position and their relationship in abduction (Figure 10) and at rest (Figure 2) should be noted.

FIGURE 10.   X-ray of the metacarpophalangeal joint of the index finger in abduction. It should be noted that the radial relationship of the articulating surfaces of the two bones is the same when the joint is at rest (Figure 2) and in flexion (Figure 4).

thumb. Figure 8 illustrates the position adopted to elicit the opening up of the lateral aspect of the joint.

The relative position of the articular surfaces of the bones when the medial aspect of the joint is tilted open is shown radiographically in Figure 9. Comparison should be made with their relative positions when the joint is abducted (Figure 10) and at rest (see Figure 2).

Rotation. The examiner maintains his grip on the head of the metacarpal bone and flexes the proximal and distal inter-phalangeal joints of the subject's finger. He grasps the distal end of the proximal phalanx between his thumb and his index and middle fingers and places his fourth finger on the other side of the subject's middle phalanx, thus crooking the subject's finger between his fingers. He then rotates the proximal phalanx clockwise and counterclockwise in its long axis, the base of this phalanx thus rotating upon the head of the metacarpal bone. Figure 11 illustrates the position adopted to elicit this movement.

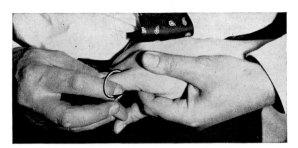

FIGURE 11.   Rotation of the base of the phalanx on the head of the metacarpal bone. Note the leverage achieved around the model's crooked index finger, ensuring that rotation is in the long axis of the phalanx.

In examining for this movement at a distal interphalangeal joint there is no way of crooking the subject's finger to produce leverage by which the movement can be elicited. In the distal interphalangeal joint the movement has to be elicited by simple rotation in the long axis, maintaining the head of the middle phalanx in the stable position.

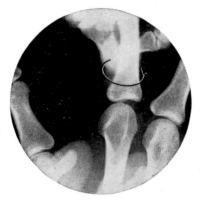

FIGURE 12. X-ray of the metacarpophalangeal joint at the limit of the joint-play movement of rotation. The relationship of the base of the phalanx to the head of the metacarpal bone is entirely different to that shown in any other of the movements illustrated in this series of x-rays.

Figure 12 illustrates the position of the base of the phalanx in relation to the head of the metacarpal bone at the completion of counterclockwise rotation in the movement of the joint play. The extent of the movement of the base of the phalanx on the head of the metacarpal bone is best appreciated when their positions are compared to those shown when the joint is at rest (see Figure 2).

5

The Hand

The Distal Intermetacarpal Joints

The movements of joint play between the heads of each metacarpal bone are: (1) anteroposterior glide and (2) rotation.
Of course, the joints between these bones are not true synovial
joints anatomically, but functionally the movement between
them may be impaired, and, if so, the symptoms of pain are
produced just as though they were synovial joints. In clinical
practice, the movements between the heads of the metacarpal
bones are seldom lost, whereas there are similar movements
between the heads of the metatarsal bones in the feet which
are frequently lost, their loss being the commonest cause of
metatarsalgia. The movements between the metacarpal heads
are more easily performed than those between the metatarsal
heads, and if these movements are understood in the hand, they
are more easily appreciated when we come to deal with the
feet.

The metacarpal bones move around the stationary axis of
the third metacarpal bone. There is no intimate movement between the heads of the first and second metacarpal bones in
the hand, in contradistinction to the most important movement
between the heads of the first and second metatarsal bones in

40

the feet. The movements of the head of the fifth metacarpal bone on the head of the fourth, in the left hand, are used to illustrate joint play of the distal intermetacarpal joints.

Anteroposterior Glide. With the subject's elbow flexed and the forearm in the neutral position, the examiner stands facing the dorsum of the hand. He grasps the neck of the fourth metacarpal bone between the fingers and thumb of the right hand and the neck of the fifth metacarpal bone between the thumb and index finger of the left hand, moving the fifth metacarpal bone forward and backward on the stabilized head of the fourth metacarpal bone. The head of the fourth metacarpal

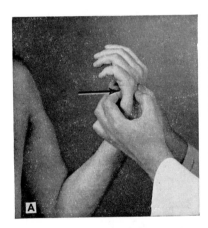 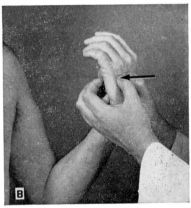

FIGURE 13A. Completion of the posterior (dorsal) phase of the anteroposterior glide of the head of the fifth metacarpal bone on the head of the fourth. The head of the fourth metacarpal bone is being stabilized by examiner's right hand.

FIGURE 13B. Completion of the anterior (volar) phase of the anteroposterior glide of the head of the fifth metacarpal bone on that of the fourth. The head of the fourth metacarpal bone is being stabilized.

bone is moved in a similar way on the stabilized head of the third metacarpal bone. Figures 13A and 13B illustrate the position adopted to elicit these movements, Figure 13A showing the completion of the dorsal movement and Figure 13B showing the completion of the volar movement. The examiner reverses the role of his hands when moving the head of the second metacarpal bone forward and backward on the stabilized head of the third metacarpal bone.

Rotation. The examiner stabilizes the fourth metacarpal bone by holding its neck between the thumb and index finger of his right hand. He then grasps the neck of the fifth metacarpal bone between the thumb and index finger of his left hand and, with a shoulder swing, rotates the head of the fifth metacarpal bone, first clockwise and then counterclockwise.

Figures 14A and 14B illustrate the position adopted to elicit

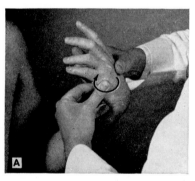 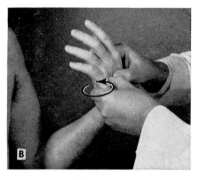

FIGURE 14A. Anterior (clockwise) rotation of the head of the fifth metacarpal bone on that of the fourth. The head of the fourth metacarpal bone is being stabilized. Compare the position of the examiner's left thumb and index finger (the mobilizing hand) with that used when performing the antero-posterior glide, as illustrated in Figures 13A and 13B.

FIGURE 14B. Posterior (counterclockwise) rotation of the head of the fifth metacarpal bone on that of the fourth. The head of the fourth metacarpal bone is being stabilized.

these movements. Figure 14A illustrates the extreme of clockwise rotation, and Figure 14B illustrates the extreme of counterclockwise rotation. The head of the fourth metacarpal bone is
moved in a similar way on the stabilized head of the third
metacarpal bone. The role of the examiner's hands is reversed
to rotate in both directions the head of the second metacarpal
bone on the stabilized head of the third metacarpal bone.

The Carpometacarpal Joints

Indirect Movement of Spread and Extension. It is almost
impossible to move the bases of the metacarpal bones on the
distal row of carpal bones, specifically. In clinical practice these
joints do lose their function, but this cannot be demonstrated
specifically except that, when the distal row of carpal bones is
tilted backward on the proximal row (see page 52), the fingers do not spread and extend as they should (see Figure 23).
Such movement as takes place at the carpometacarpal joints
is purely involuntary, and its presence or absence must be ob-
served while examination for the movements at the midcarpal
joint is being undertaken.

6

The Wrist

When it is remembered that there are sixteen synovial joints which make up the wrist, it will be realized that it is rather ingenuous to talk of a painful wrist. Fortunately, the eight carpal bones of the wrist are involved in two major functional joints, which makes our discussion of this a little simpler. Figure 15 is a schematic illustration to show these two major composite joints at the wrist. For clinical purposes the wrist may be di-

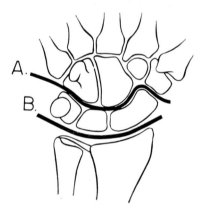

FIGURE 15. Diagrammatic illustration of the carpal bones to show the two main composite joints at the wrist. For the most part, extension occurs at the midcarpal joint (A); whereas, for the most part, flexion occurs at the radioulnocarpal joint (B).

vided into three major clinical areas: the midcarpal joint, the
radiocarpal joint, and the ulnomeniscocarpal joint. Figure 16,
an anteroposterior radiographic view of a normal left wrist,

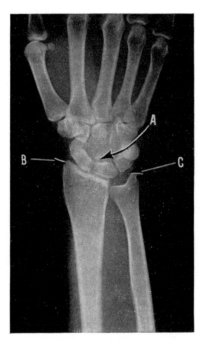

FIGURE 16.   An anteroposterior radiograph of a normal wrist. The
major clinical composite joints are indicated by arrows and designated as follows: A — the midcarpal joint, B — the radiocarpal
joint, and C — the ulnomeniscocarpal joint.

shows the position and relationship of the bones of the carpus
to each other and to the lower ends of the radius and ulna
proximally and to the bases of the metacarpal bones distally.
These relationships should be kept in mind and compared with
those at the completion of the normal joint-play movements
described and illustrated later.

Normal Voluntary Movements

For the most part, extension at the wrist takes place at the midcarpal joint, which is made up of the articular surfaces of the navicular, lunate, and triquetral bones proximally and the articular surfaces of the greater and lesser multangular, capitate, and hamate bones distally. Figure 17, a lateral radio-

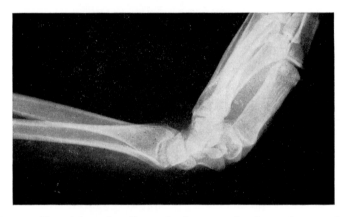

FIGURE 17.   A lateral radiograph of a normal wrist at the completion of the normal voluntary movement of extension. Note that the movement largely occurs at the midcarpal joint, designated "A" in Figures 15 and 16. Comparison should be made with Figure 18, which shows the wrist in flexion.

graphic view of a normal wrist in extension, clearly shows that this movement occurs for the most part at the midcarpal joint. Comparison should be made with Figure 18 which shows flexion at a normal wrist.

For the most part, flexion takes place at the radiocarpal joint, which is made up of the articular surface of the lower end of the radius and the articular surfaces of the navicular and the lunate bones. Figure 18, a lateral radiographic view of a nor-

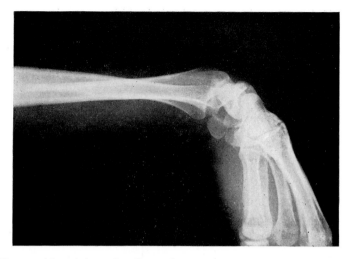

FIGURE 18. A lateral radiograph of a normal wrist at the completion of the normal voluntary movement of flexion. Note that the movement largely occurs at the radiocarpal joint, designated "B" in Figure 16. Comparison should be made with Figure 17, which shows the wrist in extension.

mal wrist in flexion, clearly shows that this movement occurs for the most part at the radiocarpal joint. Comparison should be made with Figure 17 which shows extension at a normal wrist.

The ulnomeniscocarpal (ulnomeniscotriquetral) joint is largely concerned with the function of supination and pronation of the forearm. There is one other joint at the wrist which is often overlooked, that is, the inferior radioulnar joint, which also is involved in the movements of pronation and supination.

Thus, when a patient presents himself with inability to flex his wrist or complains of pain while performing this movement, one's attention should be focused on the radiocarpal joint. If he presents himself with an inability to extend the wrist or complains of pain while attempting to perform this movement, one's attention should be focused on the midcarpal joint. Fi-

nally, if the presenting complaint is inability to supinate or pro-
nate the forearm, or of pain on attempting these movements,
one's attention should be directed at the ulnomeniscocarpal joint
and the inferior radioulnar joint. For illustration of the joint-
play movements in these joints of the wrist, the model's left
arm is being examined in most cases.

The Midcarpal Joint

The movements of joint play at this joint are: (1) long axis
extension, (2) anteroposterior glide, and (3) a backward tilt of
the distal carpal bones on the proximal carpal bones.

Long Axis Extension. With the subject's elbow flexed at a
right angle and the forearm in the neutral position between
supination and pronation, the examiner places his right hand

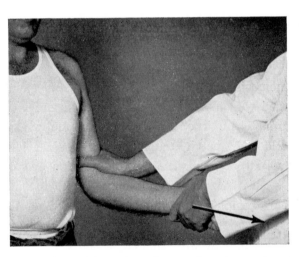

FIGURE 19. The position adopted to produce long axis extension
at the midcarpal joint. Arrow shows direction of pull used to execute this movement.

anteriorly over the condylar region of the subject's humerus at the elbow. He then grasps the wrist area with his left hand, the thumb being just distal to the radial styloid process and his index finger just distal to the ulnar styloid process where, it will be noted, there are natural indentations that prevent the thumb and finger from slipping down the hand when a pull is exerted. Figure 19 illustrates the position adopted to elicit this movement. The examiner exerts traction with his left hand, using a rotatory body swing, and stabilizes the subject's forearm by countertraction, pressure being applied with his right hand at the subject's elbow.

Anteroposterior Glide. With the subject's arm flexed at the elbow and the forearm in the neutral position, the examiner grasps the subject's wrist with his right hand so that his thumb and forefinger are placed over the proximal row of carpal bones dorsally. The examiner's wrist is extended so that his metacarpophalangeal joints rest over the long axis of the lower end of the radius. His left hand, also dorsiflexed, grasps the subject's hand so that the thumb and forefinger are placed over the distal row of carpal bones and his metacarpophalangeal line is also in the long axis of the subject's radius. The subject's wrist is just flexed. The examiner's right hand stabilizes the proximal row of carpal bones and his left hand thrusts forward in such a way that the line of force approximates the index finger of the examiner's left hand toward the index finger of his right hand at an angle of about 45 degrees. Figure 20A illustrates the position adopted to elicit this movement; Figure 20B illustrates the position at the completion of the movement; and Figure 20C, using double-exposure techniques, illustrates the range of the movement.

Figure 21, a lateral radiographic view of a normal wrist,

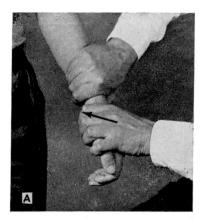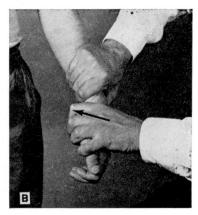

FIGURE 20A.   The position adopted to elicit the anteroposterior movement at the midcarpal joint, designated "A" in Figure 15. Note that the examiner's wrists should be dorsiflexed so that the thrusting force (in the direction of arrow) of his mobilizing left hand is parallel to the joint line.

FIGURE 20B.   The position at the completion of the anterior phase of the anteroposterior movement at the midcarpal joint. Note that the index finger of the examiner's mobilizing left hand (in the direction of arrow) has approximated toward the index finger of his stabilizing right hand.

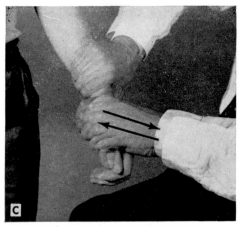

FIGURE 20C.   Double exposure illustrates the extent of the range of the anteroposterior movement at the midcarpal joint.

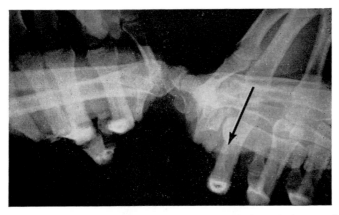

FIGURE 21. The midcarpal joint at the completion of the anterior phase of the joint-play movement of anteroposterior glide. Arrow at right shows direction of thrust.

shows the midcarpal joint at completion of the anterior phase of the anteroposterior glide joint-play movement (see Figure 20B). The extent of the movement would be greater had it been technically possible to make the exposure with the forearm held in the neutral position instead of in a considerable degree of pronation. However, if one compares this picture with Figure 32 (a lateral view of the normal wrist at rest), on page 63, there can be no doubt that the normal joint-play movement of anteroposterior glide occurs at the midcarpal joint.

This achieves the anterior phase of the anteroposterior glide; the posterior phase is achieved when the thrust is released and the rebound into the neutral position occurs. It should be noted that anteroposterior glide cannot be demonstrated with the subject's forearm in full supination or full pronation, and that the extent of the movement increases to a maximum as the subject's forearm is rotated from one or another extreme into the neutral midposition.

Backward Tilt of the Distal Carpal Bones on the Proximal Carpal Bones. With the subject's arm flexed at the elbow and

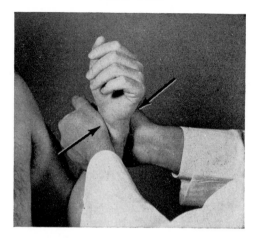

FIGURE 22. The position of the examiner's hands to perform the joint-play movement of backward tilt of the distal carpal bones on the proximal carpal bones. The performance of this movement depends upon the accurate placement of the examiner's thenar eminences over the correct bones.

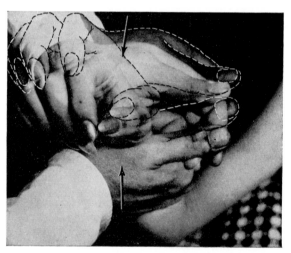

FIGURE 23. In this double exposure the natural outlines of the examiner's hands and the model's right hand at rest are in the starting position to perform the joint-play movement of backward tilt of the distal carpal bones on the proximal carpal bones, as illustrated

the forearm held in the vertical and neutral position, the examiner places the thenar eminence of his left hand on the volar aspect of the proximal row of carpal bones and the thenar eminence of his right hand on the dorsal aspect of the distal row of carpal bones, clasping his fingers around the radial aspect of the subject's wrist. The examiner dorsiflexes his wrists so that the long axis of his radii are directed at right angles to the subject's carpus. The examiner then squeezes his hands to-

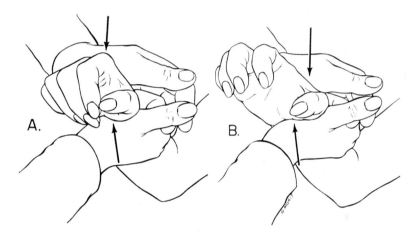

FIGURE 24A.   Tracing from Figure 23 of the position of the examiner's hands and model's right hand placed to produce the joint-play movement of backward tilt of the distal carpal bones on the proximal carpal bones.

FIGURE 24B.   Tracing from Figure 23 of the position of the examiner's hands and the model's right hand at the completion of the joint-play movement of backward tilt of the distal carpal bones on the proximal carpal bones. Note the extension and the spreading of the model's fingers, which take place only when this joint-play movement is elicited correctly.

in Figure 22. The inked-in outlines are the positions of the examiner's hands and the model's hand at the completion of this movement. Figures 24A and 24B are tracings of each of these positions separated.

gether, thrusting together his thenar eminences in the long axis of his radii. This movement tilts the subject's distal row of carpal bones backward upon the proximal row of carpal bones, particularly the capitate on the navicular end lunate, tilting the anterior aspect of the midcarpal joint open. The capitate tilts backwards.

Figure 22 illustrates the position adopted to achieve this movement. Figure 23, by double exposure, illustrates the extent of the movement, in this case the right hand of the model being shown. The extension and spread of the model's fingers should be noted. These finger movements of the model's hand on completion of the movement are the only demonstrable criteria that the midcarpal joint movement has been properly accomplished. Figures 24A and 24B are tracings taken from the two exposures of Figure 23 and show the extension and spread of the fingers when the movement is properly performed.

The Intercarpal Joints

Forward and Backward Shift. There is, of course, a range of movement between each carpal bone. This cannot be readily appreciated on clinical examination unless there has been a traumatic subluxation of one of the bones upon another. This most commonly happens in the wrist when the lunate bone subluxes backward on its adjacent carpal bones. The range of specific involuntary movement is probably such that each bone can just move forward and backward upon its neighboring bones.

The Radiocarpal Joint

The radiocarpal joint is the composite joint between the distal end of the radius and the navicular and lunate bones. The movements of joint play at this joint are: (1) long axis extension, (2) backward tilt of the navicular and lunate bones on the lower end of the radius, and (3) side tilt of the navicular on the radius.

Long Axis Extension. Long axis extension at this joint is achieved in exactly the same manner as long axis extension at the midcarpal joint.

With the subject's elbow fixed at a right angle and the forearm in the midposition, the examiner places his right hand anteriorly over the condylar region of the subject's humerus at the elbow. He then grasps the wrist area with his left hand, the thumb being just distal to the radial styloid process and his index finger just distal to the ulnar styloid process where, it will be noted, there is a natural indentation that prevents the thumb and finger from slipping down the hand when a pull is exerted. The examiner exerts traction with his left hand, using a rotatory body swing, while he stabilizes the forearm by countertraction,

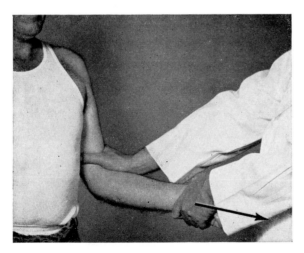

FIGURE 25. The position adopted to produce long axis extension at the radiocarpal joint. Arrow shows direction of pull by examiner.

applying pressure with his right hand at the subject's elbow. Figure 25 illustrates the position adopted to elicit this movement.

Backward Tilt of the Navicular and Lunate Bones on the Radius. The examiner stands facing the subject with the latter's arm flexed at the elbow and the forearm pronated. The examiner places his right thumb over the dorsal aspect of the navicular, the thumb being in the long axis of the subject's radius; he places his left thumb over the lunate, again the thumb being in the long axis of the subject's radius. The examiner then crooks his index fingers around the wrist so that they lie at right angles to his thumbs, but on the volar surface; their tips are placed over the navicular and the lunate in such a manner that the examiner is grasping the navicular with his right hand, and

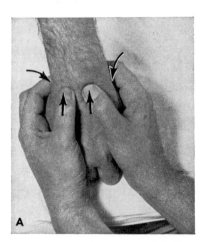

FIGURE 26A. The position of the examiner's hands to elicit the backward tilt of the navicular and lunate bones upon the lower end of the radius. The examiner's right thumb and index finger grasp the navicular; the examiner's left thumb and index finger grasp the lunate. Figure 26B is a lateral view of the same position.

the lunate with his left hand (see Figures 26A, B). The navicular and the lunate are gently flexed forward on the lower end of the radius as the forearm is being gently raised by slightly increasing flexion at the elbow. The forearm is then whipped downward toward the floor by sudden ulnar deviation of the examiner's wrists, the movement being arrested in such a way

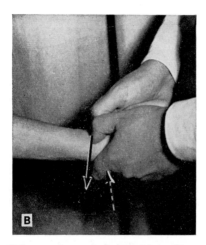

FIGURE 26B. Side-on view of the position illustrated in Figure 26A, in which the examiner is grasping the model's navicular and lunate bones prior to eliciting their backward tilt upon the lower end of the radius. Arrows show line of force used by examiner to evoke joint-play movements.

that, momentarily, the navicular and lunate are tilted backward on the lower end of the radius, which tilts the radiocarpal joint open at its volar aspect.

Side Tilt of the Navicular on the Radius. The examiner grasps the lower end of the radius and ulna between the thumb and index finger of his right hand and the proximal row of carpal bones between the thumb and index finger of his left hand, holding the subject's arm in the neutral position and flexed at the elbow. Using his thumbs as a pivot, the examiner stabilizes the lower end of the forearm bones with his right hand, and, by ulnar deviation of his left wrist, he tilts the navicular away from the lower end of the radius. The position adopted to elicit this movement is shown in Figure 27A. An alternate method

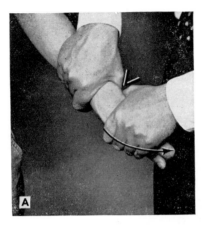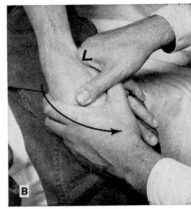

FIGURE 27A.   Joint-play movement of side tilt of the navicular away from the radius. The examiner's right hand stabilizes the lower end of the radius, and with both thumbs used as a pivot, the navicular is tilted away from the lower end of the radius when the examiner turns his left hand into ulnar deviation.

FIGURE 27B.   Alternate method of tilting the navicular away from the lower end of the radius. The examiner uses the index finger of his right hand as a pivot at the ulnomeniscocarpal joint and pulls the model's hand into ulnar deviation with his left hand.

of achieving the same movement of joint play is illustrated in Figure 27B. Figure 28 is an x-ray taken at the completion of the joint-play movement of side tilt of the navicular on the lower end of the radius. The extent of this movement may be seen if one compares the relationship of these two bones in this figure with that when they are at rest (see Figure 16).

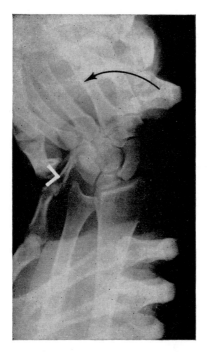

FIGURE 28. Radiograph showing the completion of the joint-play movement of side tilt of the navicular away from the radius.

The Ulnomeniscotriquetral Joint

The movements of joint play at the ulnomeniscocarpal (ulno-meniscotriquetral) joint are: (1) long axis extension, (2) anteroposterior glide, and (3) side tilt.

Long Axis Extension. Long axis extension is achieved in the same manner as that at the midcarpal joint and the radiocarpal joint. With the subject's elbow flexed at a right angle and the forearm in the midposition, the examiner places his right hand anteriorly over the condylar region of the humerus at the subject's elbow and grasps the wrist area with his left hand, the thumb being just distal to the radial styloid process and his index finger just distal to the ulnar styloid process where, it will be noted, there is a natural indentation that prevents the thumb and finger from slipping down the hand when a pull is exerted. The position adopted to elicit this movement is shown in Figure 29. The examiner exerts traction with his left hand, using a

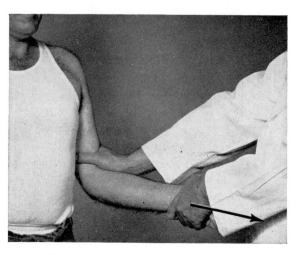

FIGURE 29.   The position adopted to produce long axis extension at the ulnomeniscocarpal joint. Arrow shows direction of pull used to execute this movement.

rotatory body swing, and stabilizes the forearm by countertraction by applying pressure with his right hand at the elbow.

Anteroposterior Glide. With the subject's arm flexed at the elbow and the forearm held in the vertical and neutral position, the examiner holds the radial half of the subject's hand in his right hand. He then places his left thumb over the posterior aspect of the neck of the lower end of the ulna, the thumb being at right angles to the long axis of the ulna. He next crooks his left index finger and places its proximal interphalangeal joint over the pisiform bone on the volar aspect of the subject's wrist. The examiner then pinches his left thumb and index finger together, thereby carrying the lower end of the subject's ulna forward on the triquetrum as the triquetrum moves backward on the lower end of the ulna and the meniscus which lies between them. Figure 30 illustrates the position adopted to elicit the

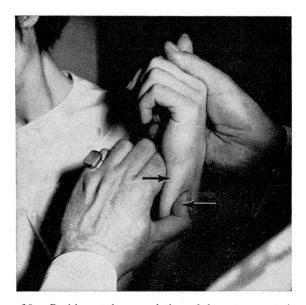

FIGURE 30. Position at the completion of the anteroposterior glide of the ulna on the triquetrum (between which lies a meniscus) in its anterior phase. The posterior phase is achieved on rebound from this position. Note the examiner's right hand merely stabilizes the model's left hand and arm. The movement by the examiner is achieved by pinching his left thumb and forefinger together in parallel.

movement, the photograph being taken at the completion of it.

Figure 31, a lateral radiographic view of a normal wrist, shows the ulnomeniscocarpal joint at the completion of the anterior

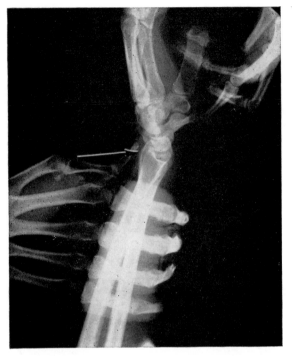

FIGURE 31. The joint between the lower end of the ulna and the triquetral bone (ulnomeniscotriquetral joint) toward the completion of the joint-play movement of anterior glide.

phase of the normal joint-play movement of anteroposterior glide. For clarity, the examiner's index finger is not hooked over the pisiform bone, which prevents this movement from being carried to its fullest extent. The movement of anteroposterior glide at the ulnomeniscocarpal joint is better appreciated if Figure 31 is compared with Figure 32, a lateral x-ray view of a normal wrist at rest. Figure 32 should also be compared with Figure 21, again better to appreciate the nature of the joint-play movement of anteroposterior glide at the midcarpal joint.

Side Tilt of the Triquetrum on the Ulna. The examiner grasps the lower ends of the radius and ulna between the thumb and in-

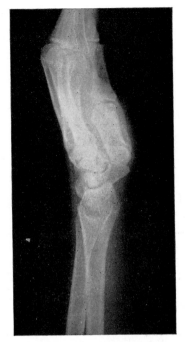

FIGURE 32. A lateral radiographic
view of a normal wrist.

dex finger of his right hand and the proximal row of carpal
bones between the thumb and index finger of his left hand, holding the subject's arm in the neutral position and flexed at the
elbow. Using his index fingers as a pivot, the examiner stabilizes
the lower end of the forearm bones with his right hand and tilts
the subject's hand into radial deviation with his left hand. Figure
33 demonstrates the position adopted to elicit this movement at
the end of the movement. An alternate way of achieving the same
movement is shown in Figure 34.

The Inferior Radioulnar Joint

The movements of joint play at this joint are: (1) anteropos-

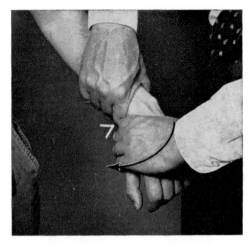

FIGURE 33.   Side tilt of the triquetrum away from the ulna and the
meniscus upon which it rests. The examiner's right hand stabilizes
the lower end of the ulna, and with both index fingers used as a
pivot, the triquetrum is pulled away from the lower end of the ulna
when the examiner swings his left hand into radial deviation.

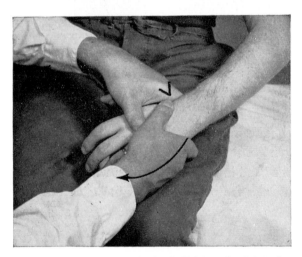

FIGURE 34.   An alternate method of eliciting the joint-play movement of side tilt at the ulnomeniscotriquetral joint. The examiner
uses the index finger of his left hand as a pivot at the radiocarpal
joint and pulls the model's hand into radial deviation with his right
hand, thus tilting the triquetrum away from the lower end of the
ulna and the meniscus upon which it rests.

terior glide and (2) rotation of the lower end of the ulna on the radius.

Anteroposterior Glide. With the subject's arm flexed at the elbow and the forearm held in the vertical and neutral position, the examiner places his right thumb posteriorly over the neck of the lower end of the radius, the thumb being at right angles to the long axis of the radius, and crooks his index finger around the wrist so that it lies anteriorly with the proximal phalanx at right angles to the radius and the distal phalanges in the long axis of the radius. He places his left thumb over the neck of the lower end of the ulna posteriorly with it at right angles to the long axis of the ulna and crooks his index finger around the wrist

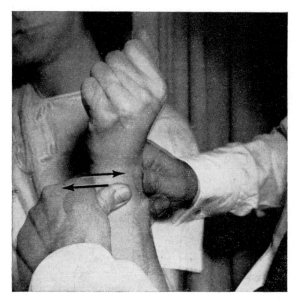

FIGURE 35. The position adopted to elicit the anteroposterior glide at the inferior radioulnar joint. The examiner stabilizes the lower end of the radius with his right hand and pushes the lower end of the ulna forward upon it with his left hand. The double exposure indicates the range of this movement.

so that its proximal phalanx is at right angles to the long axis of the ulna anteriorly and the distal phalanges are in its long axis. The examiner stabilizes the lower end of the radius with his right hand and alternately pushes the lower end of the ulna forward and backward upon it. Figure 35 illustrates the position adopted to elicit this movement, and the double exposure indicates the extent of the range anteriorly.

Rotation. Using the same examining position as described for eliciting the joint-play movement of anteroposterior glide at this joint (see Figure 35), the examiner now wings his forearms at right angles to the subject's forearm. Again, stabilizing the lower

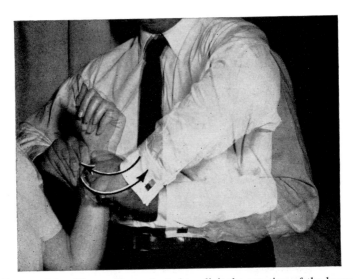

FIGURE 36.   The position adopted to elicit the rotation of the lower end of the ulna on the lower end of the radius at the inferior radio-ulnar joint. The double exposure illustrates the extent of the move-ment, and the examiner's shoulder swing should be particularly noted. The difference of this movement and that of the anteropos-terior glide is clearly seen in this illustration, when compared with Figure 35.

end of the radius with his right hand, the examiner rotates the lower end of the subject's ulna on the radius, using a swing of his left shoulder girdle forward and backward.

Figure 36 illustrates the position adopted to elicit this movement, the double exposure indicating the extent of the movement and emphasizing the swing of the shoulder girdle used to achieve the movement.

7

The Elbow

The elbow is another limb area which, by usage, is called a joint and yet in which there are three major joints, each with their own range of movement and each of which must be considered as a separate entity. These joints are the superior radio-ulnar joint, the radiohumeral joint, and the humeroulnar joint. The left arm is used in most cases for illustration.

The Superior Radioulnar Joint

The movements of joint play at this joint are: (1) upward glide of the head of the radius on the ulna, (2) downward glide of the head of the radius on the ulna, and (3) rotation of the head of the radius on the ulna, which is independent of supination and pronation of the forearm.

Upward Glide of the Head of the Radius. To examine for this joint-play movement the examiner places the palm of his dorsiflexed right hand over the posterior aspect of the lower end of the subject's humerus. With his elbow flexed to a right angle, the examiner places the thenar eminence of the palm of his dorsiflexed left hand over the thenar eminence of the subject's dorsiflexed hand, with the subject's and his thumbs inter-

68

twined. The examiner's two radii and the subject's radius are thus all in one straight line (Figure 37). The examiner stabilizes

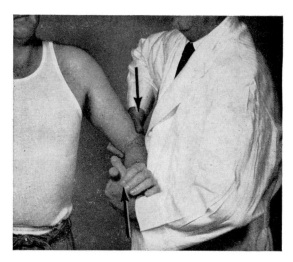

FIGURE 37. The position adopted to elicit the upward glide of the head of the radius on the ulna at the superior radioulnar joint. The examiner's two radii and the model's radius are all in line. The arrows show line of force applied by the examiner; the examiner's right hand stabilizes model's arm while the examiner's left hand is mobilizing the model's radius.

the subject's arm with his right hand and thrusts along the long axis of the subject's radius with his left hand.

Downward Glide of the Head of the Radius. The downward glide of the head of the radius on the ulna is tested for in exactly the same manner as the movement of long axis extension at the midcarpal, radiocarpal, and ulnomeniscotriquetral joints. With the subject's elbow flexed at a right angle and his forearm in the midposition, the examiner places his right hand over the anterior aspect of the inferior condylar region of the subject's humerus at the elbow. With his left hand the examiner grasps the wrist area, his thumb being just distal to the radial styloid process and his index finger just distal to the ulnar styloid process, the natural indentations at these points preventing the thumb and finger from slipping down the hand when a pull is exerted. The examiner exerts traction with his left hand, using a rotatory body swing, and stabilizes the forearm by counter-traction with pressure by his right hand at the elbow. Figure 38 illustrates the position adopted to elicit this movement.

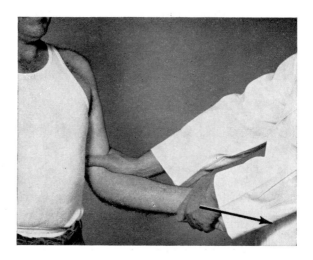

FIGURE 38.   The position adopted to elicit the downward glide of the head of the radius on the ulna at the superior radioulnar joint. The examiner's left hand is the mobilizing hand.

Rotation of the Head of the Radius on the Ulna. With the subject in the recumbent supine position, and his arm in full supination, the examiner places the thenar eminence of his right hand over the anterior aspect of the head of the radius. With his left hand he grasps the subject's wrist with his thumb on its dorsal aspect and his fingers over its ventral aspect. Figure 39A shows the position of the examiner's hands relative to the sub-

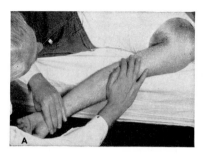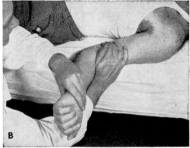

FIGURE 39A. The position adopted at the beginning of the examination of a normal joint-play movement of rotation of the head of the radius on the ulna. This figure must be considered serially with Figures 39B, 39C, and 39D. Note that this examination is carried out with the subject in a recumbent position.

FIGURE 39B. Photograph showing the increase in the carrying angle of the elbow as the arm is being positioned to examine for rotation of the head of the radius on the ulna. Full supination of the model's forearm must be maintained.

ject's arm at the beginning of this movement. Maintaining both the subject's upper arm in this starting position and his own right thenar eminence over the head of the subject's radius, the examiner, with his left hand, increases the carrying angle at the subject's elbow, at the same time maintaining the forearm in full supination. Figure 39B illustrates this movement.

At the point where the carrying angle of the subject's elbow is maximum, the examiner then brings the subject's elbow into flexion while still maintaining the forearm in full supination until the examiner feels the head of the radius firmly pressing up against his right thenar eminence (Figure 39C). At this point, maintaining the subject's arm rigidly in this position, the examiner whips the subject's forearm into full pronation, thus rotating the head of the radius backward on the ulna. Figure 39D, which should be compared with Figure 39C, shows the subject's arm in the same angle of flexion at the elbow, but now with his forearm in full pronation. Figure 40 shows with the use of a

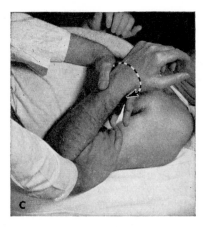

FIGURE 39C. The final position achieved before the head of the
radius is rotated upon the ulna by pronating the forearm. The head
of the radius should be felt impinging upon the thenar eminence of
the examiner's right hand.

double exposure how this movement is achieved without moving
the relative position of the subject's upper and lower arm in
flexion when it is pronated.

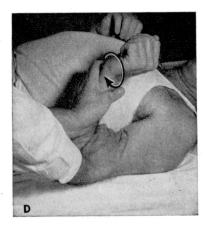

FIGURE 39D. Position at the completion of the normal joint-play
movement of rotation of the head of the radius on the ulna at the
superior radioulnar joint.

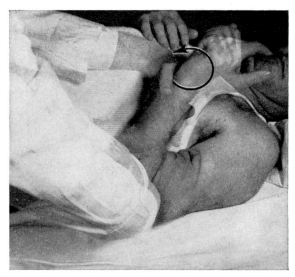

FIGURE 40. This double exposure illustration shows how the forearm is taken from supination into pronation without altering the angle of flexion at the elbow. It is during this examining movement that the head of the radius rotates upon the ulna at the superior radioulnar joint.

The Radiohumeral Joint

The specific movement that takes place between the articular surface of the head of the radius upon the capitulum of the humerus is one of a change of radial relationship as the elbow is flexed and then extended, and this movement is specifically an involuntary one in all its phases. Its presence and its loss is fundamentally dependent upon the normal function of the superior radioulnar joint. Dysfunction of the radiohumeral joint results from dysfunction in the superior radioulnar joint and can only be corrected by restoring movement to the latter joint. The exception to this is when there is a meniscus present within the joint.

Intra-articular Meniscus Lock. In about 10 per cent of people there is an intra-articular meniscus in this joint, which may
cause symptoms of pain and dysfunction on movement of the
joint in the same manner as the menisci do in the knee joint.
It must be assumed that, when this happens, the meniscus loses
its functional anatomical relationship to the articular surfaces of
the humerus and the radius. To detect this mechanical dysfunction, the examiner grasps the subject's upper arm over the posterior aspect of the condyles of the humerus with his right hand,
the thumb resting over the head of the subject's radius anterolaterally. With his left hand the examiner grasps the wrist over
its posterior aspect and then flexes the elbow fully, pronates the
forearm fully, and flexes the wrist fully. Figure 41A illustrates
this position before the start of the examining movement. The
examiner now extends the elbow, the completion of the extension

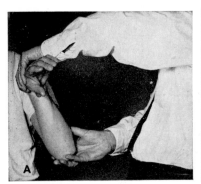 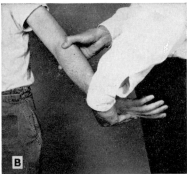

FIGURE 41A.   The position adopted at the beginning of the movement which determines whether there is a meniscal block at the
radiohumeral joint. The examiner's right thumb is placed over the
head of the radius anterolaterally. The full pronation of the forearm
and full flexion of the wrist should be noted.

FIGURE 41B.   The examining movement started in Figure 41A is
now completed. The examiner's right thumb remains in position
over the head of the radius, and his right hand has stabilized the
upper arm throughout the movement. His left hand has extended the
forearm, maintaining it in full pronation and the wrist in full flexion.

movement being shown in Figure 41B. If there is a meniscal block at the radiohumeral joint (dysfunction), as the extensor muscles tighten toward the end of this extension movement (full pronation of the forearm and full flexion of the wrist being maintained at all times), the patient feels pain, and the movement becomes resisted as though the joint were locking. It may be that an infolding of the synovium is acting as a meniscus.

The Humeroulnar Joint

This joint lies between the trochlea of the humerus and the olecranon of the ulna. The coronoid process of the ulna moves into the coronoid fossa of the humerus on full flexion and the

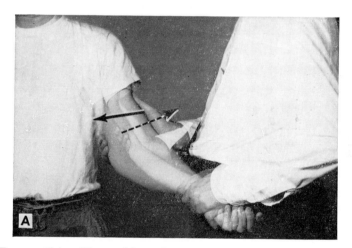

FIGURE 42A. The position adopted by the examiner to perform in the upright position the joint-play movements of medial and lateral tilt of the olecranon away from the long axis of the forearm. The examiner's left hand, which grasps the model's wrist across its volar surface, is the stabilizing hand. The extent of the movement with the elbow flexed at about 15 degrees is indicated by the double exposure; its extent lessens as the arm is extended by the examiner's right hand during the examining movement. Figure 42B illustrates the position of the mobilizing hand with the model in the proper position of recumbency in which the examination should be performed.

olecranon process of the ulna moves into the olecranon fossa of the humerus on full extension. The movement of joint play at this joint is one of a medial and lateral tilt of the ulna away from the long axis of the humerus. Pain from loss of this movement may result from the olecranon process' pinching the synovial fat pad as it attempts to enter the olecranon fossa askew.

Medial and Lateral Tilt of the Olecranon. To elicit this movement, which is absent of course in full extension, the examiner flexes the subject's elbow about 15 degrees. With his left hand, which acts as the stabilizer, he grasps the subject's wrist across its volar aspect. He then grasps the lower end of the subject's humerus posteriorly with his right hand, his thumb being on the lateral aspect of the subject's upper arm. The examiner then exerts alternately a medial and lateral thrust on the lower

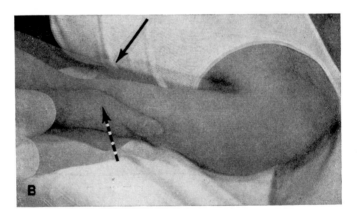

FIGURE 42B.   The position of the examiner's mobilizing right hand during the joint-play movements of medial and lateral tilt at the humeroulnar joint with the subject in the recumbent position. The examiner carries the lower end of the humerus, first medially and then laterally. The ulnar olecranon "grinds" into its fossa in the humerus as the arm is extended by raising the lower end of the humerus at the same time.

end of the humerus with his right hand while at the same time lifting the subject's elbow into extension. Figure 42A illustrates the position adopted to elicit this movement with the subject in a standing position, although the examination can only be achieved in a controlled manner when the subject is lying down in the supine position. The extent of this movement is less well seen when the proper examining position (Figure 42B) is used. In this latter position, the examiner also extends the elbow by lifting the lower end of the humerus as he "grinds" the ulnar olecranon into its fossa.

Reciprocally, there is a similar movement of joint play as the coronoid process of the ulna is received into the coronoid fossa of the humerus when the arm is fully flexed, but clinically this cannot be distinguished and, to all intents and purposes, can be disregarded.

8

The Shoulder

Though only two bones take part in formation of the shoulder joint (glenohumeral joint) itself, movement of it is dependent upon the synchronous normal movement of three other joints — the acromioclavicular, the sternoclavicular, and the scapulo-chest wall joints. The last, of course, is not a synovial joint, but for functional purposes it acts as one in that the scapula may become bound down on the chest wall by disuse, direct trauma, myostatic contractures or fibrositis of the muscles attached to it, or immobilization, in which case the function of the glenohumeral joint is impaired.

The Glenohumeral Joint

The movements of joint play at this joint are: (1) lateral movement of the head of the humerus away from the glenoid cavity; (2) anterior movement of the head of the humerus within the glenoid cavity; (3) posterior shear of the head of the humerus within the glenoid cavity; (4) downward and backward movement of the head of the humerus within the glenoid cavity; (5) outward and backward movement of the head of the humerus within the glenoid cavity; (6) direct posterior movement of the head of the humerus within the glenoid cavity with the arm forward flexed at 90 degrees (90-degree posterior movement of the head of the humerus); and (7) external rotation of the head of the humerus within the glenoid cavity. It should be noted here that whereas the voluntary movement of the glenohumeral joint, for the most part, tends to raise the arm upward, almost all the movements in the range of joint play are directed at pulling the head of the humerus downward and only one — the sixth joint-play movement mentioned above — requires movement of the subject's arm from the side of his body to any extent.

The examination for all the movements of joint play at the glenohumeral joint are done with the patient in the recumbent supine position. The shoulder must be supported by the examining table but right at the edge of it so that, in performing the movements, the examiner does not have to abduct the arm when adopting the examining positions. The left glenohumeral joint is used for illustration.

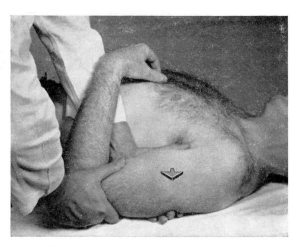

FIGURE 43. The position adopted to push the head of the humerus laterally away from the glenoid cavity. The subject's arm is adjacent to his chest wall. The examiner's left hand acts as the mobilizer; his right (stabilizing) hand just lifts the arm into the neutral position.

Lateral Movement of the Head of the Humerus away from the Glenoid Cavity. The examiner's left hand is placed on the medial aspect of the upper end of the subject's upper arm just beneath the axilla. His right hand is placed on the posterolateral aspect of the subject's elbow, with the latter's forearm resting across his body and being supported by the examiner's left forearm (Figure 43). The examiner's right (stabilizing) hand exerts pressure to hold the subject's arm at his side, while the examiner's left (mobilizing) hand thrusts outward laterally to move the head of the humerus laterally away from the glenoid cavity.

Anterior Movement of the Head of the Humerus within the Glenoid Cavity. The position of the examiner's hands to elicit this movement is basically the same as that described above except that his left hand is moved medially around the subject's upper arm so that it is posterior to the upper end of the humerus.

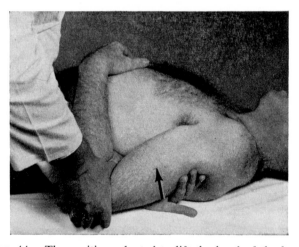

FIGURE 44. The position adopted to lift the head of the humerus forward within the glenoid cavity. Note the marked range of gross movement anteriorly of the forequarter, the slack of which has to be taken up before the joint-play movement is elicited,

The examiner's stabilizing right hand at the elbow now exerts pressure toward the couch while his left hand lifts the subject's upper arm upward away from the couch, the head of the humerus moving forward within the glenoid cavity. Figure 44 illustrates the position adopted to elicit this movement. Since there is a large range of gross movement anteriorly in the fore-quarter, the slack of this movement has to be taken up before the examining movement to elicit the movement of joint play is made.

Posterior Shear of the Head of the Humerus within the Glenoid Cavity. To elicit this movement the examiner reverses the position of his hands; his left hand is now placed on the posterior aspect of the subject's elbow, the latter's forearm resting

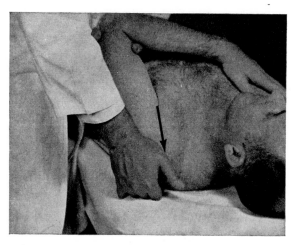

FIGURE 45. The position adopted to shear the head of the humerus backward within the glenoid cavity. Note the examiner's left hand lifts the elbow through perhaps 10 degrees of flexion of the arm to take up the slack before stabilizing it. The examiner applies the thrust (arrow) used to elicit the movement through his right thenar eminence, which is placed over the greater tuberosity of the model's humerus.

82   JOINT PAIN

across his forearm, and his right hand is placed so that the thenar eminence is directly over the greater tuberosity of the subject's humerus. The examiner's left hand raises the subject's arm through a few degrees until it is felt that the scapula is firmly against the couch, at which point a thrust is made into the couch by the examiner's right hand, shearing the head of the humerus backward within the glenoid cavity. Figure 45 illustrates the position adopted to elicit this movement; the examiner's left hand having raised the subject's arm a few degrees to take up slack.

Downward and Backward Movement of the Head of the Humerus within the Glenoid Cavity. The examiner crouches

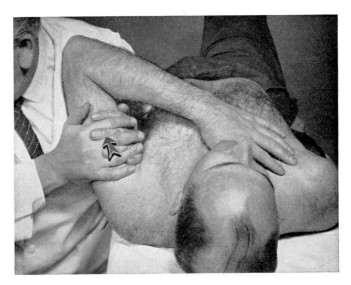

FIGURE 46.   The position adopted to elicit the downward and backward glide of the head of the humerus within the glenoid cavity. The pull by the examiner's hands is along the line of the edge of the couch; the subject's arm must not be abducted. The examiner thrusts upward with his shoulder in a counterarc to take up the additional slack which results from the movement of the head of the humerus within the glenoid cavity.

down so that the shawl area of his left shoulder can be placed as a fulcrum at the lower end of the subject's humerus posteriorly. The examiner's two hands are clasped together over the anterior aspect of the surgical neck of the subject's humerus; the subject's arm is forward flexed — in a normal subject to about 45 degrees, while in a patient to the angle just before which pain is appreciated. The head of the humerus is then pulled downward and backward within the glenoid cavity, and as the movement occurs, the examiner thrusts upward with his shoulder in a counterarc to take up the slack of the movement of the arm which is produced by the movement of the head of the humerus. It should be noted that the examiner does not attempt to forward flex the arm as he does it. Figure 46 illustrates the position adopted to elicit this movement.

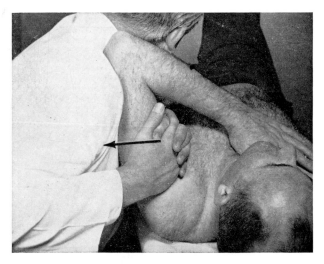

FIGURE 47. The position adopted to elicit the outward and backward joint-play movement of the head of the humerus within the glenoid cavity. The examiner thrusts upward with his shoulder in a counterarc to take up the additional slack which results from the movement of the head of the humerus within the glenoid cavity.

Outward and Backward Movement of the Head of the Humerus within the Glenoid Cavity. The examiner now turns to face the subject in such a position that the latter's arm now rests comfortably on the shawl area of the examiner's right shoulder. In this position the examiner's right shoulder acts as a fulcrum at the lower third of the subject's humerus. The examiner then clasps his hands over the medial aspect of the surgical neck of the humerus and pulls it away from the glenoid cavity and backward within it. The examiner thrusts his shoulder forward in a counter-arc to take up the slack of the movement of the arm which is produced by the movement of the head of the humerus. The position adopted to elicit this movement is shown in Figure 47. It should be noted that the examiner does not attempt to thrust the subject's arm across his body.

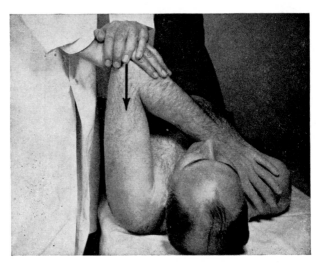

FIGURE 48. The position adopted to elicit the direct posterior movement of the head of the humerus backward within the glenoid cavity. Note this movement can only be achieved if the model's arm is forward flexed to 90 degrees.

Ninety-Degree Posterior Movement of the Head of the Humerus within the Glenoid Cavity. The examiner remains in the same position in relation to the subject, whose arm is forward flexed to a right angle — in a patient, to the angle at which limitation is noted. The examiner places both hands directly over the elbow and thrusts downward into the couch, thus moving the head of the humerus backward within the glenoid cavity. Figure 48 illustrates the position adopted to elicit this movement.

External Rotation of the Head of the Humerus within the Glenoid Cavity. The subject's arm is kept in the rest position at

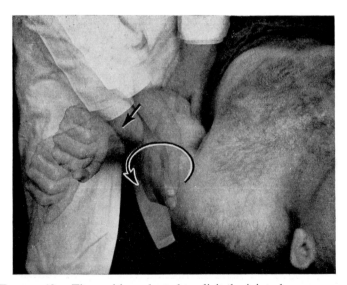

FIGURE 49. The position adopted to elicit the joint-play movement of rotation of the head of the humerus within the glenoid cavity. Note that the starting position is at the end of the voluntary excursion of external rotation. The examiner's left hand stabilizes the elbow, and it is his right hand which rotates the shaft of the humerus. The dorsal aspect of his wrist lies upon the model's forearm, pressing slightly downward on it, assisting the rotation movement. The double exposure illustrates the additional range of external rotation because of the joint-play movement.

his side. The elbow is lifted sufficiently to avoid the position of extension which is normally adopted when one is lying down in the supine position. The examiner's left hand grasps the subject's elbow, which is flexed. With his right hand he clasps the subject's upper arm in the region of the surgical neck of the humerus posteriorly. This necessitates dorsiflexing his wrist so that the subject's forearm is beneath his forearm. The external rotation movement of joint play is primarily effected by rotation of the humeral shaft but is aided to a minimal degree by a rotatory force imparted through the forearm. Before the joint-play movement is elicited, the subject's arm has to be taken through its possible range of voluntary external rotation which takes up the slack in the joint and it is at this point, when all of the slack is taken up, that the examiner further rotates the head of the humerus outward within the glenoid cavity to achieve the joint-play movement. Figure 49 illustrates the position adopted to elicit this movement, and the double exposure illustrates the extent of the joint-play movement of external rotation beyond the limit of voluntary external rotation.

Movements of the Clavicle

To allow the glenohumeral joint to move freely, the clavicle has to rotate on its own axis, and to achieve full extension of the arm above the head in normal voluntary movement. This rotation has to be 50 degrees. Thus, any limitation of movement at the acromioclavicular or sternoclavicular joints impairs freedom of voluntary movement at the glenohumeral joint. It will be realized that all movement at the acromioclavicular and sternoclavicular joints is involuntary movement in that the clavicle cannot be rotated upon its axis by the use of voluntary muscles.

Equally, one cannot produce this rotatory movement by manipulative means. There is, however, movement in the range of joint play that can be elicited at each joint, the absence of which will prevent the normal rotation of the clavicle. It should be remembered that there is an intra-articular cartilage in the sternoclavicular joint which may become loose or detached and interfere with normal movement of this joint.

The Acromioclavicular Joint

Anteroposterior Glide. Movement of joint play in the acromioclavicular joint is that of an anteroposterior (superoinferior)

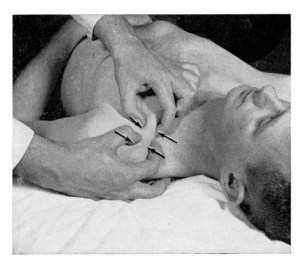

FIGURE 50. The position adopted to elicit the joint-play movement at the acromioclavicular joint — which is an anteroposterior shear of the clavicle upon the acromion. The examiner's grasp upon the clavicle is on its outer third and the direction of movement approaches the horizontal. Comparison should be made with the similar grasp upon the clavicle in Figure 51, where the movement is more vertical as the sternoclavicular joint is moved.

shear in a somewhat horizontal plane. To elicit this, the examiner grasps the clavicle between his thumbs and index fingers at the junction of its middle and outer thirds and carries it forward and backward through the anteroposterior range (Figure 50).

The Sternoclavicular Joint

Anteroposterior Glide. The movement of joint play in this joint is that of an anteroposterior (superoinferior) shear in a somewhat vertical plane. To elicit this, the examiner grasps the clavicle between his thumbs and index fingers at the junction of its inner and middle thirds and carries it upward and downward through the anteroposterior range (Figure 51).

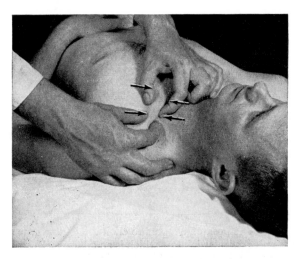

FIGURE 51. The position adopted to elicit the anteroposterior shear at the sternoclavicular joint. The examiner grasps the medial third of the clavicle, the direction of movement approaching the vertical.

The Scapula-Chest Wall Junction

For free movement of the glenohumeral joint, the scapula has to rotate upon the chest wall through an arc of about 60 degrees. This scapular rotation is an involuntary movement in that it cannot be performed alone either by the use of voluntary muscles or without moving the glenohumeral joint.

Scapular Rotation. To elicit the involuntary movement of rotation of the scapula on the chest wall, the subject lies in the lateral position. With his left hand the examiner then grasps the point of the subject's shoulder over the acromion process, and with his right hand he grasps the dependent angle of the scapula. When the subject is relaxed, the scapula can be made

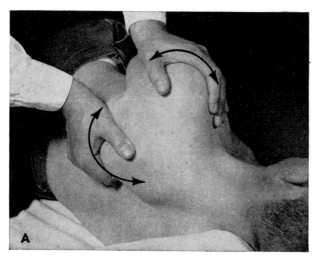

FIGURE 52A.   The position adopted to elicit the rotatory movement of the scapula upon the chest wall. In this case both hands mobilize the scapula.

to wing sufficiently for the examiner to get the tips of his fingers beneath it. The winged angle of the scapula is then swung downward and outward, while the tip of the shoulder is swung upward and inward, the scapula thus being rotated upon the chest wall. Figure 52A illustrates the position adopted to elicit this movement; Figure 52B, with its double exposure, illustrates the extent of the movement.

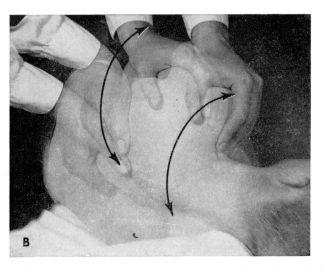

FIGURE 52B. This double exposure illustrates the extent of the range of joint-play rotation of the scapula upon the chest wall.

9

The Toes

The Metatarsophalangeal and Interphalangeal Joints

The range of joint play in the metatarsophalangeal joints and the interphalangeal joints is the same as that described for the small joints of the fingers, though the extent of each movement is different and the facility with which they may be performed is less because of the anatomical structure of the soft parts of the foot. Fortunately, in clinical practice, one is usually limited to treatment of the metatarsophalangeal joints, since the digital joints of the toes seldom are involved in pain-producing dysfunction.

The metatarsophalangeal joint of the big toe is used to illustrate the range of joint-play movement in all these joints. The movements of joint play at this joint are: (1) long axis extension, (2) anteroposterior tilt, (3) side tilt medially and laterally, and (4) rotation.

Long Axis Extension. The examiner holds the head of the metatarsal bone between the thumb and the index finger of his right hand and grasps the base of the proximal phalanx between the thumb and index finger of his left hand, the thumb being placed on the dorsal aspect and the index finger being placed on the plantar aspect. He then pulls the proximal phalanx away from the head of the metatarsal bone in the direction of the long axis of the toe. The position adopted to perform this movement is shown in Figure 53.

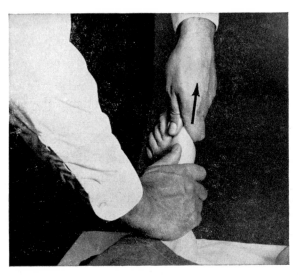

FIGURE 53.   Position used to elicit the joint-play movement of long axis extension at the metatarsophalangeal joint of the big toe. Note the golf-club grip by the examiner's left hand and stabilization of the head of the metatarsal by his right hand. Arrow shows direction of pull.

Anteroposterior Tilt. The examiner maintains the grip upon the head of the metatarsal bone with his right hand and places the tip of his left thumb just distal to the base of the proximal phalanx dorsally and the tip of his left index finger just distal to the base of the phalanx on its plantar surface. Using the left thumb and the left index finger alternately as a fulcrum, the examiner tilts the base of the subject's phalanx alternately backward and forward, opening either the dorsal or the plantar aspect of the joint. The posterior phase of this joint-play movement, as well as the position adopted to elicit it, is shown in Figure 54. There is actually a mobilizing force in both finger and thumb in each movement.

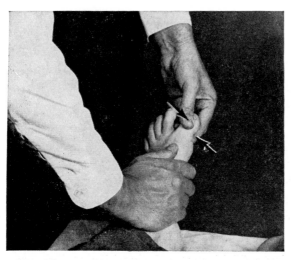

FIGURE 54. The posterior tilt at the completion of the posterior phase of the anteroposterior tilt at the metatarsophalangeal joint. Note the examiner's left index finger being used as a pivot (lower arrow) on the plantar aspect of the proximal phalanx, while the thumb presses forward (upper arrow) over it.

Side Tilt Medially and Laterally. The examiner maintains his grip on the head of the metatarsal bone with his right hand. He places the tip of his left thumb deep in the web between the first and second toes and the tip of the left index finger medially just distal to the base of the proximal phalanx. Using the thumb as a pivot, the metatarsophalangeal joint is tilted open on its medial aspect by exerting pressure through the tip of the left index finger, using the tip of the left thumb as a fulcrum. Then, using the tip of the index finger as a pivot, the metatarsophalangeal joint is tilted open laterally by exerting pressure through the

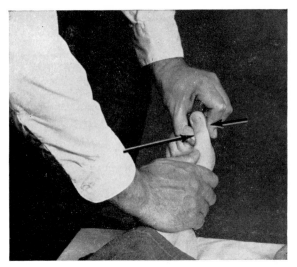

FIGURE 55.   The position at the completion of the joint-play movement of side tilt laterally, opening up the medial aspect of the metatarsophalangeal joint. Note the examiner's left thumb is being used
as a pivot, while the index finger tilts the base of the phalanx laterally on the metatarsal bone.

thumb. Figure 55 illustrates the position at the completion of
the medial phase of the joint-play movement of side tilt as well
as the position adopted to elicit this movement. There is actually
a mobilizing force in both finger and thumb in each movement.

Rotation. The examiner maintains his grip on the head of
the metatarsal bone with his right hand. The interphalangeal
joint of the big toe is flexed. The examiner then grasps the proximal phalanx with his left thumb and index and middle fingers,
and hooks the distal phalanx of his fourth and fifth fingers on
the lateral aspect of the subject's distal flexed phalanx. Alternately, the examiner rotates the proximal phalanx on the metatarsal
head clockwise and counterclockwise in its long axis. The position adopted to elicit this movement is shown in Figure 56.

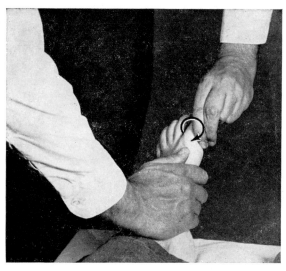

FIGURE 56. Rotation of the base of the phalanx on the head of the metatarsal bone. The model's distal phalanx is flexed and the distal phalanx of the examiner's fourth and fifth fingers are on its lateral aspect. The leverage is thus achieved that ensures that rotation is in the long axis of the proximal phalanx.

The joint-play movements of the other metatarsophalangeal joints and the interphalangeal joints are elicited in the same way, only the degree of normal movement being different.

10

The Foot

The Distal Intermetatarsal Joints

The movements of joint play between the heads of each meta-tarsal bone are: (1) anteroposterior glide and (2) rotation. Of course, the joints between these bones are not true synovial joints anatomically, but functionally the movement between them may be impaired; if so, dysfunction occurs and the symptoms of pain are produced just as though they were synovial joints. It will be remembered that a similar range of movement has been described between the heads of the metacarpal bones of the hands, and it was pointed out that the metacarpal heads move around the stationary axis of the third metacarpal bone. In the foot, however, the stationary axis is the second metatarsal bone. With this exception, the movements to be elicited are the same as those already described for the metacarpal heads in the hand (Chap. 5, page 41).

Anteroposterior Glide. With the subject in the recumbent position, the examiner sits at the end of the couch, facing the plantar aspect of the subject's foot. (The left foot is used for illustration.) The examiner grasps the neck of the second meta-tarsal bone, his right thumb being on the plantar aspect and his fingers on the dorsal aspect of it. He grasps the metatarsal bone of the first toe in a similar manner with his left hand. The second metatarsal bone is stabilized, and the head of the first metatarsal bone is moved upward and downward upon it. The reader should remember that the words *upward* and *downward* are used in an anatomical sense but that the movement of the heads of the metatarsal bones is positionally *forward* and *backward*.

The role of the examiner's hands is then reversed and he grasps the second metatarsal bone with his left hand and with his right (mobilizing) hand moves the head of the third metatarsal bone upward and downward upon it. He then stabilizes the third metatarsal bone with his left hand and with his right hand moves the head of the fourth metatarsal bone upward and downward upon it. Finally the fourth metatarsal bone is stabilized with the examiner's left hand and the head of the fifth

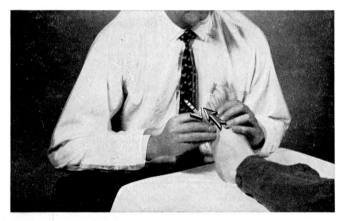

FIGURE 57. The joint-play movement of anteroposterior glide of the head of the fifth metatarsal bone on the head of the fourth. The double exposure illustrates the range of the dorsal (posterior) phase of the joint-play movement. (It must be remembered that the second metatarsal bone is the axis in the foot, whereas the third metacarpal bone forms the axis in the hand.)

metatarsal bone is moved upward and downward upon it. The movement of the head of the fifth metatarsal bone upon the head of the fourth is shown in Figure 57.

Rotation. The examiner stabilizes the head of the second metatarsal bone in the same way that has been described above in the examination to elicit the joint-play movement of antero-posterior glide. He then grasps the neck of the first metatarsal bone between his left thumb and index finger, which are now placed at right angles to the long axis of the metatarsal bone. With a shoulder swing, he rotates the head of the first metatarsal bone clockwise and counterclockwise upon the head of the second metatarsal bone.

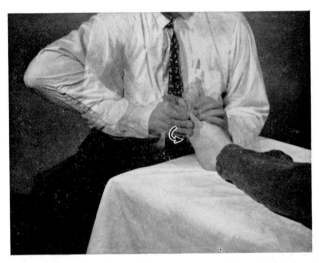

FIGURE 58. The joint-play movement of rotation of the head of the fifth metatarsal bone upon the head of the fourth. The double exposure illustrates the range of the dorsal (counterclockwise) part of the movement and also the use of the shoulder swing to achieve it. The difference between this rotation movement and the antero-posterior glide is best appreciated by comparing the position of the examiner's right (mobilizing) arm and hand in this figure with their positions in Figure 57.

The role of the examiner's hands is then reversed, and his left hand now stabilizes the second metatarsal bone. The neck of the third metatarsal bone is grasped between the examiner's right thumb and index finger, placed at right angles to its long axis, and with a shoulder swing, he rotates it clockwise and counterclockwise on the stabilized head of the second metatarsal bone. The examiner then stabilizes the third metatarsal bone with his left hand, and with his right hand he rotates the head of the fourth metatarsal bone on the head of the third. The examiner finally stabilizes the fourth metatarsal bone and rotates the head of the fifth metatarsal bone on the head of the fourth. Figure 58 illustrates the position adopted to produce this last movement, the double exposure showing the extent of the movement.

The Tarsometatarsal Joints

As with the carpometacarpal joints of the hands, movements of the tarsometatarsal joints are all in the involuntary range. There are also facets between the bases of the metatarsal bones which are, in fact, part of the synovial joints. Joint-play movements at the tarsometatarsal joints and proximal intermetatarsal joints are: (1) anteroposterior glide and (2) rotation.

Anteroposterior Glide. The distal tarsal bones are grasped in relation to the base of the metatarsal bones. The bases of the metatarsal bones are grasped over their dorsal aspect by the examiner's right hand, while his left hand stabilizes the distal tarsal bones. His mobilizing right hand alternately thrusts dorsally and plantarward, performing an anteroposterior glide movement (superoinferior in direction) between the bases of the metatarsal bones and the adjacent tarsal bones. Figure 59 illustrates this movement. The base of the fifth metatarsal bone can

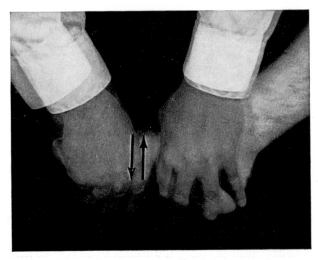

FIGURE 59.   The position adopted to elicit the joint-play movement
of anteroposterior glide at the joints between the bases of the metatarsal bones and the distal row of the tarsal bones. The double exposure indicates the range of movement plantarward. The thumb
and index finger of the examiner's left (stabilizing) hand must carefully be positioned over the cuneiform bones and the cuboid bone
so that movement is not mistakenly elicited at the midtarsal joint, as
illustrated in Figure 61. The examiner's right hand is the mobilizing
hand.

be moved independently on the cuboid bone to elicit the anteroposterior glide specific to this joint.

Rotation. There is a different degree of rotation of the bases
of the metatarsal bones on their adjacent tarsal bones, and the
movement cannot specifically be elicited at each joint but has
to be performed at all of the joints at once. Using the right foot
for illustration, the tarsus is stabilized by grasping it over its
dorsal aspect with the left hand. The examiner faces the lateral
aspect of the foot. He then cradles the necks of the metatarsal
bones between his right thumb, which is placed across them
dorsally, and the four fingers, which are placed across them on

their plantar surface. The examiner then rotates the forefoot as a whole, first into eversion and then into inversion. This produces a rotation of the bases of the metatarsal bones upon the tarsal bones, first clockwise and then counterclockwise. Figure 60 illustrates the position adopted to elicit this movement, the double exposure showing the extent of the clockwise movement.

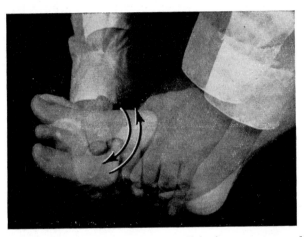

FIGURE 60.   The position adopted to elicit the movement of rotation of the bases of the metatarsal bones on the distal row of tarsal bones. The double exposure indicates the clockwise (eversion) part of this movement; a similar range is obtainable in the counterclockwise (inversion) direction. The thumb and index finger of the examiner's left (stabilizing) hand must be carefully positioned over the distal tarsal bones so that the joint-play movement is limited to the tarso-metatarsal joints.

The Midtarsal Joints

Anteroposterior Glide. There are no true voluntary movements of the midtarsal joints, but there is one important involuntary movement upon which the resilience of the foot to take up the stresses and strains of function largely depends, that is, an anteroposterior (superoinferior) type of movement of the distal cuneiform bones on the navicular (scaphoid), and the navicular upon the talus. Using the left foot for illustration, the examiner stabilizes the navicular and talus with his right hand over their dorsal aspect and grasps the three cuneiform bones with his left hand and moves them dorsally and plantarward alternately. He then releases his grip on the navicular by placing his hand further back toward the mortise joint and grasps the navicular and cuboid bone with his left (mobilizing) hand; he alternately exerts a dorsal and plantar movement of them on the stabilized talus and calcaneus (Figure 61) eliciting an antero-

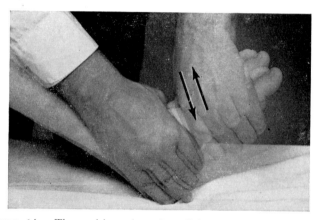

FIGURE 61.   The position adopted to elicit the joint-play movement of anteroposterior glide at the midtarsal joint. The double exposure indicates the range of movement plantarward. The thumb and index finger of the examiner's right (stabilizing) hand must carefully be positioned to grasp proximally to the articulating surfaces of the talus and calcaneus. The thumb and index finger of his mobilizing left hand must carefully be positioned over the navicular and cuboid to avoid movement being achieved at the wrong joint.

posterior movement. The anteroposterior movements of the navicular on the talus and the cuboid on the calcaneus are well elicited by the examining maneuver which is used to elicit long axis traction at the subtalar (subastragaloid) joint (page 110). Figure 68 (page 111) shows radiographically the extent to which the navicular and the cuboid move.

The Intertarsal Joints

Forward and Backward Shifts. There is, of course, a range of movement (superoinferior in direction) between each tarsal bone. This cannot be appreciated clinically on examination unless there has been a traumatic subluxation of one of the bones upon another. The subluxation is usually dorsalward, and there is a clinical sign of pain on pressing the affected bone plantarward on examination. The range of the specific involuntary movement probably consists of each bone's moving slightly upward and downward upon its neighboring bones.

11

The Ankle

The Mortise Joint

The mortise joint is made up of the lower tibial condyle and the tibial and fibular malleoli, which constitutes one joint aspect, and the superior aspect of the talus (astragalus). There are but two movements of joint play at this joint: (1) long axis extension and (2) anteroposterior glide. The right foot is used for illustration.

Long Axis Extension. The examiner sits on the couch with his back to the subject, whose hip is abducted and flexed to not less than 90 degrees and whose knee is also flexed to a right angle. He grasps the lower leg around the ankle, the left thenar web being placed posteriorly to the Achilles tendon and the right thenar web being placed over the dorsum of the foot as close to the ankle as possible. The examiner then leans backward on the subject's thigh, while he pushes the foot away from him in the long axis of the lower leg, maintaining the foot at right angles to it. Figure 62 illustrates the position adopted for the examining maneuver, and the double exposure shows the extent of the movement of long axis extension.

Anteroposterior Glide. With the subject recumbent and the hip, knee, and ankle all at a 90-degree angle, the examiner

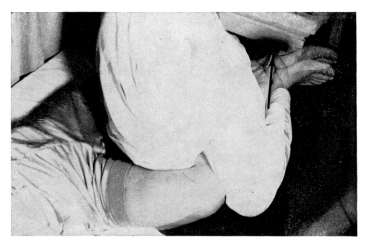

FIGURE 62. The position adopted to elicit the joint-play movement of long axis extension at the mortise joint. Note the hip, knee, and ankle are held at right angles. The examiner thrusts forward in the long axis of the tibia, exerting countertraction by leaning backward against the posterior aspect of the model's thigh. Note the thrust of the examiner's hands is through the web between his thumbs and index fingers, and there is no true grip on the sides of the model's foot by them. The double exposure illustrates the extent of the joint-play movement of long axis extension.

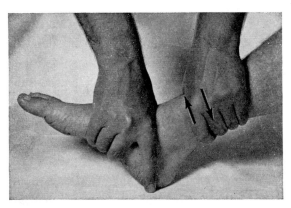

FIGURE 63. The position adopted to elicit the anteroposterior glide of the articulating surfaces of the tibia and fibula on the talus. The examiner's left hand is the mobilizing hand. Note that the foot is held at right angles to the lower leg by the examiner's right (stabilizing) hand; the model's knee and hip are flexed.

grasps the subject's lower leg around the ankle just above the malleoli with his left hand; he grasps the dorsum of the foot with the right hand, which will stabilize it during the performance of this movement. The mobilizing left hand then pulls forward and pushes backward alternately, thereby moving the mortise forward and backward upon the immobile superior talar facet. The position adopted for eliciting this movement is shown in Figure 63.

The Subtalar (Subastragaloid) Joint

Anatomy texts describe this joint simply as the joint between the talus and the calcaneus whose range of movement is that of inversion and eversion at the ankle. In fact, the function of this joint is far from simple; its most important movement, which is seldom described, is a rocking movement of the talus upon the calcaneus which is entirely independent of voluntary muscle action. It is this movement that takes up all the stresses and strains of stubbing the toes and that spares the ankle from gross trauma, both at toe-off and at heel strike in the normal function of walking and when abnormal stresses that tend to twist the ankle to a great extent are inflicted at the ankle joint. If it were not for this involuntary rocking motion at the subtalar joint, fracture dislocations around the ankle would be commonplace.

Differentiation of Movement from the Mortise Joint. The importance of clinical differentiation of mortise-joint pain from subtalar-joint pain cannot be too highly stressed. This differentiation is quite easily achieved, however. With the subject recumbent and the hip, knee, and ankle all at right angles, the examiner grasps the lower leg some 6 inches above the malleoli

with his left hand and supports the sole of the foot with his right
hand. The subject's foot is now resting upon the postero-inferior
angle of the calcaneus, and the examiner rocks the foot on it by
pushing upward and downward on the tibia, thereby producing
plantar flexion and dorsiflexion of the foot at the mortise joint.
If these movements are full, free, and painless, there is obviously
no pathological condition in this joint. The position adopted for
these examining maneuvers and the normal range of voluntary
movement at the mortise joint are shown in Figure 64.

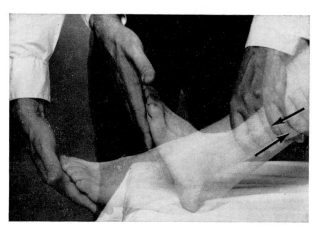

FIGURE 64.   The examining position adopted to elicit pure dorsiflexion and plantar flexion of the mortise joint. The double exposure
illustrates the extent of this voluntary movement. The examiner's left
hand elicits the movement of rocking the foot on the postero-inferior angle of the calcaneus. The examiner's right hand simply maintains the sole of the foot in its unchanging plane.

Talar Rock. To examine for the normal rocking movement
at the subtalar joint, instead of stopping the plantar-flexion
movement at its limit, the examiner now pushes through the
limit of this movement, thereby producing the rock of the talus
on the calcaneus. This movement is not one of hyperflexion

plantarward which, if performed, simply puts an abnormal stretch upon the anterior transverse ligament of the ankle joint and produces pain; such pain simply indicates that an abnormal movement is being performed at the mortise joint. The subtalar rock is produced as the thrust of the examiner's hand down the tibia is resisted by friction where the calcaneus is resting on the couch. This friction force is sufficient to stabilize the cal-

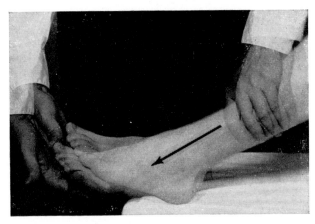

FIGURE 65.   The additional movement of apparent plantar flexion that is obtained when the talar rock is brought into play. The examiner thrusts down the long axis of the tibia with his left hand (arrow) through the limit of plantar flexion which was illustrated in Figure 64. The double exposure shows how the foot slips slightly forward on the couch, indicating that this is not forced plantar flexion. The examiner's right hand is simply used as a guide.

caneus while the talus rocks forward upon it. The range of the talar rock beyond full plantar flexion at the mortise joint is shown in Figure 65. Pain on the performance of this movement indicates some pathological condition giving rise to pain in the subtalar joint. Figure 66 is a lateral radiographic view of a normal ankle, and the appearance of the subastragaloid joint

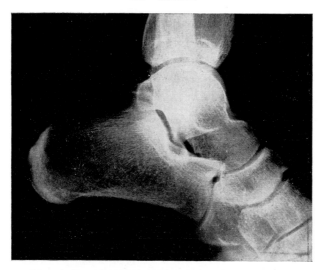

FIGURE 66. A lateral radiographic view of a normal ankle joint. The appearance of the subtalar (subastragaloid) joint should be kept in mind when studying the illustrations (Figures 68, 70A, and 70B) of joint-play movement at this important joint.

should be noted and compared with its appearance when the movements of joint play are being elicited (Figures 70A and 70B, page 114).

The stress of inversion or eversion of the foot may be added while performing this movement if the examiner keeps the sole of the foot in the horizontal plane with his supporting hand and exerts a lateral or medial thrust upon the subject's lower leg, using his left forearm, during the performance of this movement. Further clinical evidence of pathology in the subtalar joint is obtained by noting that maximum tenderness is elicited on palpating through the sinus tarsi and that localized swelling is situated in relationship to this area rather than tenderness and swelling being in relationship to the fibular malleolus and the fibular collateral ligament.

The joint-play movements, then, at the subtalar joint are:

(1) long axis extension, (2) rock of talus on calcaneus, (3) side tilt medially, and (4) side tilt laterally.

Long Axis Extension. The examiner adopts the examining position that has already been described for eliciting the joint-play movement of long axis extension at the mortise joint. Long axis extension at the subtalar joint cannot be performed without exerting long axis extension at the mortise joint. In eliciting this movement, then, one deliberately breaks one of the cardinal rules of manipulative technique in that two movements are performed at the same time. Figure 67 illustrates the position adopted for eliciting the movement of long axis extension, the double exposure indicating the extent of the movement elicited. The extent of the movement illustrated, of course, is the summa-

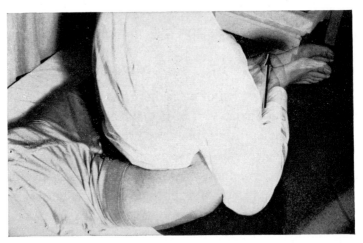

FIGURE 67. The position adopted to elicit the joint-play movement of long axis extension at the subtalar joint is exactly the same as that in Figure 62, which illustrates long axis extension at the mortise joint. The extent of the range of this movement is, of course, a summation of long axis extension at both the mortise and the subtalar joints.

tion of long axis extension at the mortise joint and at the sub-talar joint.

Figure 68 is a lateral radiographic view of a normal ankle at

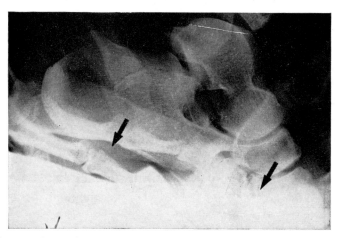

FIGURE 68.   The subtalar (subastragaloid) joint at the completion of the joint-play movement of long axis extension. The arrows indicate the direction of the thrusts of the examiner's hands.

the completion of the joint-play movement of long axis extension at the subastragaloid joint. Clearly long axis extension cannot be elicited at this joint without exerting long axis extension at the mortise joint also. The extent of this movement at the mortise joint is well illustrated, too. This situation is, of course, not unique. If the reader refers back to the topical chapters on the upper extremity, it will be noted that a similar situation is found when the movement of long axis extension is being elicited at the midcarpal joint, the radioulnocarpal joints, and when the head of the radius is being pulled downward on the ulna (see Figures 19, 25, and 38).

It is interesting to note the joint-play movements of the cuboid on the calcaneus and of the navicular on the talus which are elicited during the performance of long axis extension at the subtalar joint. It is analogous to an anteroposterior glide, the posterior phase of which occurs on the rebound when the examining stress is released. These movements were alluded to in the discussion of the joint play at the intertarsal joints (see page 103).

Rock of Talus on Calcaneus. The previous description of the talar rock was limited to its examination while the foot and ankle are in function. The examination for this specific rocking movement is now described. The position adopted by the examiner is the same as that used for eliciting the movement of long axis extension. In reproducing the joint-play movement of talar rock, it is again necessary to perform two joint-play movements at the same time because the talar rock cannot be performed

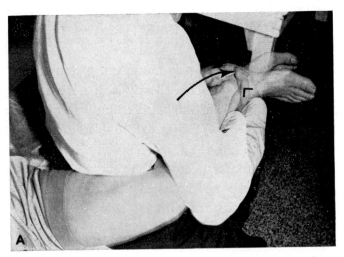

FIGURE 69A. The extent of the forward movement of the calcaneus on the talus, which is the posterior phase of the talar rock. Note the movement is elicited while full long axis extension at the mortise and subtalar joints is maintained. The examiner's left hand acts as the mobilizer (arrow), pressure being exerted on the posterior aspect of the calcaneus by the web between the thumb and index finger.

passively unless the joint is in the position of long axis extension.

Holding the foot and leg with the subtalar and mortise joints in the position of the limit of long axis extension, the examiner now pushes upward and forward with the hand which is behind the Achilles tendon, thereby rocking the calcaneus forward on the talus (Figure 69A). Then, the examiner pushes backward and downward with the hand that is on the anterodorsal aspect of the foot to produce the posterior rock of the calcaneus on the talus (Figure 69B). Figures 70A and 70B are x-rays taken at the completion of the forward phase and the backward phase of the talar rock. Figure 70A corresponds to the foot illustrated in Figure 69A; Figure 70B corresponds to the foot in Figure 69B.

These movements have nothing to do with the movements of

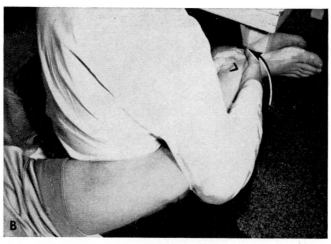

FIGURE 69B. The extent of the backward movement of the calcaneus on the talus which is the anterior phase of the talar rock. Note the movement is elicited while full long axis extension at the mortise and subtalar joints is maintained. The examiner's right (mobilizing) hand is exerting pressure indirectly on the anterior aspect of the calcaneus through the other tarsal bones by the web between the thumb and index finger.

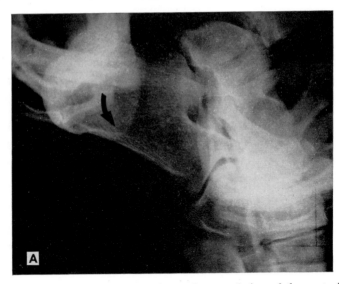

FIGURE 70A.   The subtalar joint at the completion of the posterior phase of the talar rock. The arrow indicates the direction of the thrust of the examiner's hand over the posterior aspect of the cal- caneous. The movement corresponds with that shown in Figure 69A.

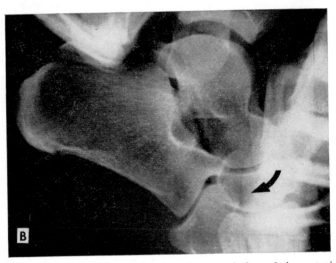

FIGURE 70B.   The subtalar joint at the completion of the anterior phase of the talar rock. The arrow indicates the direction of the thrust of the examiner's hand indirectly through the other tarsal plantar flexion and dorsiflexion, which must be studiously avoid-ed. This rocking movement of the subtalar joint is best appreciated by feeling it and by comparing the feeling of it with that of the dorsiflexion and plantar-flexion movements that take place at the mortise joint.

Side Tilt Medially. Again, the position adopted to elicit this movement is the same as that described for the previous movements and again one of the rules of manipulation technique is deliberately broken as more than one movement is performed at a time. The tilting movement, both medially and laterally, can only be achieved when the joint is at the limit of long axis extension. So, to elicit the movement of side tilt medially, first long axis extension is performed, as illustrated in

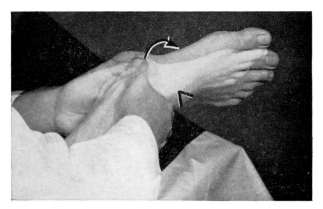

FIGURE 71. The movement of side tilt medially of the calcaneus upon the talus which tilts open the subtalar joint on its medial aspect. Note the movement is elicited while full long axis extension at the mortise and subtalar joints is maintained, as in Figure 67. The thrusting force (arrow) is through the examiner's thumbs on the medial aspect of the calcaneus. His fingers laterally are used as a pivot. The double exposure illustrates the extent of the movement.

bones over the anterior aspect of the calcaneus. This movement corresponds with that illustrated in Figure 69B.

Figure 67. When long axis extension is achieved, the examiner's thumbs, which are placed on the medial aspect of the calcaneus, thrust laterally upon the calcaneus, tilting the subtalar joint open on its medial aspect. This movement is that of a pure tilt of the calcaneus upon the talus and is not simple eversion of the foot at the subtalar joint. The extent of this movement is shown in Figure 71.

Side Tilt Laterally. This movement is elicited in exactly the same way as the movement of the side tilt medially, but in-

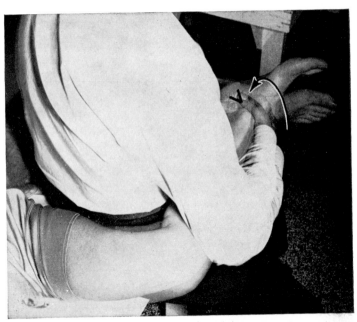

FIGURE 72. The movement of side tilt laterally of the calcaneus upon the talus, which opens up the joint on its lateral aspect. Note the movement is elicited while full long axis extension at the mortise and subtalar joints is maintained, as in Figure 67. The thrusting force is through the fingers of both hands of the examiner on the lateral aspect of the calcaneus; medially the thumbs are used as a pivot. The double exposure illustrates the extent of the movement.

stead of the tilting thrust being imparted through the thumbs on the medial aspect of the calcaneus, the tilting thrust is imparted through the fingers which are placed over the lateral aspect of the calcaneus. Figure 72 shows the extent of this movement.

12

The Knee

There are three main joints at the knee: the femorotibial joint, the patellofemoral joint, and the superior tibiofibular joint. The latter two usually receive but scant notice in clinical medicine; yet, one of the most painful "knees" I have seen was due to dysfunction in the superior tibiofibular joint, although the more usual site of pain resulting from dysfunction of this joint is in the lateral aspect of the mortise joint.

The Femorotibial Joint

The confusing thing about this joint is that the movements of joint play are known to all in that they are used to test the ligamentous and muscular stability of the joint. But if the joint is unstable, the movements are exaggerated. The importance of the normal degree of movement in each test remains unrecognized; yet, without this normal degree of movement, voluntary knee-joint movement is impaired and painful. These joint-play movements at this joint are: (1) side tilt medially, (2) side tilt laterally, (3) anteroposterior glide, and (4) rotation. In the following examinations the left knee in most cases is used for illustration.

Side Tilt Medially. The examiner grasps the thigh with his right hand posterior to the femoral condyles. The knee is un-

locked by flexing it two or three degrees. The examiner stabilizes the lower leg by grasping it around the anterior aspect of
the ankle with his left hand. Then the fermoral condyles are
thrust medially from their lateral aspect. This tilts open the
medial aspect of the joint. The position adopted to elicit this
joint-play movement is shown in Figure 73, the picture being
taken with the joint tilted open on its medial aspect.

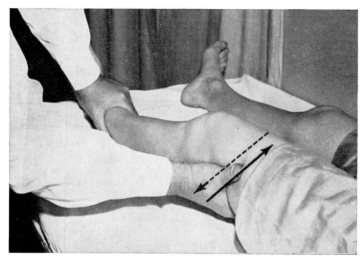

FIGURE 73. The position adopted to elicit the movement of side
tilt medially, which opens up the medial aspect of the knee joint.
The examiner's left hand stabilizes the lower leg. His right hand,
which grasps the femoral condyles, thrusts (direction of solid arrow)
from the lateral aspect of the femoral condyles, tilting the joint open
medially. Note that knee joint is slightly flexed.
To elicit side tilt laterally the examiner's hands remain in the same
position, but the thrust (direction of broken arrow) is made from
the medial aspect of the femoral condyles.

Figure 74 is an x-ray taken at the completion of the joint-
play movement of medial side tilt, as illustrated in Figure 73.
It is important to note that this is not a stress film taken with

the knee in extension to indicate dissolution of the medial collateral ligament. The knee in this illustration is unlocked in minimal flexion and the opening up of the medial aspect of the joint is the normal extent of the normal joint-play movement.

If the knee were not unlocked by minimal flexion, this would be the same test as that used to determine the integrity of the medial collateral ligament, for with the knee in full extension it is impossible to tilt the joint open medially if the medial collateral ligament is intact. Equally, if the vastus medialis muscle is weakened for some reason, the quadriceps mechanism that locks the joint is impaired, and an abnormal side tilting medially may occur. It should be remembered that the vastus me-

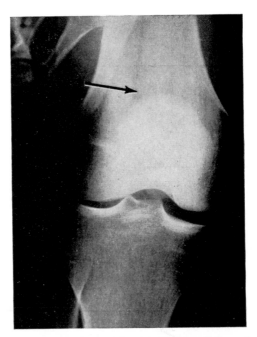

FIGURE 74. The right knee joint at the completion of the joint-play movement of side tilt medially, opening up the medial aspect of the joint. Arrow shows direction of examining thrust.

dialis muscle atrophies early in the presence of any pathological process involving the knee joint.

Side Tilt Laterally. The examiner's hands remain in the same position to elicit this movement (see Figure 73), but the thrust to tilt open the joint laterally is made from the medial aspect of the femoral condyles after the joint has been unlocked by flexing it two or three degrees. It is impossible to tilt the joint open laterally with the knee in full extension, if the lateral collateral ligament is intact; therefore, if one fails to unlock the joint, one will be determining the integrity of the lateral collateral ligament.

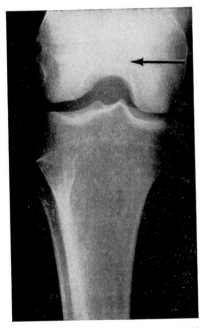

FIGURE 75. The right knee joint at the completion of the joint-play movement of side tilt, opening up the lateral aspect of the joint. Arrow indicates direction of examining thrust.

Figure 75 is an x-ray taken at completion of the joint-play movement of lateral side tilt. Again, because the knee joint is unlocked by minimal flexion, this tilting open of the lateral joint space is the extent of a normal movement and has nothing to do with the determination of the integrity of the lateral collateral ligament. Figures 74 and 75 should be compared with Figure 76, an x-ray of a normal knee joint at rest, in order better to appreciate the extent of the medial and the lateral tilts.

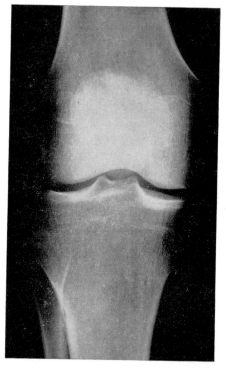

FIGURE 76.   An anteroposterior radiographic view of a normal right knee joint.

Anteroposterior Glide. These movements are best demonstrated with the knee in about 45 degrees of flexion. The exam-

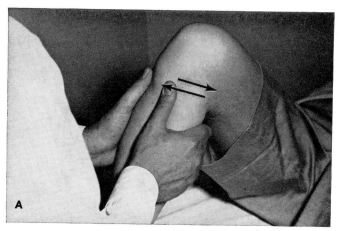

FIGURE 77A. The position adopted to elicit the joint-play movement of anteroposterior glide at the right knee joint. The examiner stabilizes the model's leg by sitting on the foot and uses both hands to produce the movement.

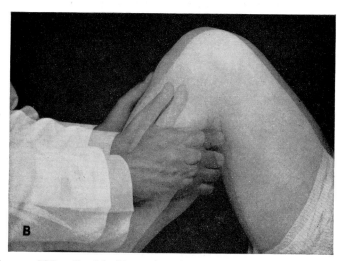

FIGURE 77B. In this illustration the extent of the normal joint-play movement is indicated by the movement of the thumbs rather than by that of the fingers which is exaggerated because of soft tissue compression.

iner sits on the subject's foot and grasps the lower leg at its proximal end, having his thumbs longitudinally in the parapatellar tendon troughs. The fingers of the examiner's hands encircle the lower leg. The tibial condyles are then pulled forward and pushed backward on the femoral condyles, which are positionally immobilized. Figure 77A shows the position adopted to elicit these movements, whereas in Figure 77B the double exposure indicates the range of normal movement in the anterior phase of the examination.

This, of course, is the manner in which the drawer sign is performed, which tests the integrity of the cruciate ligaments. But if either cruciate ligament is torn, the normal movement is exaggerated. The movements may also be exaggerated in the presence of a weakened quadriceps femoris.

The range of the normal anteroposterior movement of joint play varies with the degree of flexion at the joint. It is minimal with the knee both in extension and in full flexion, and maxi-

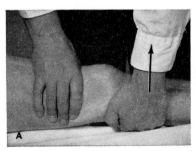
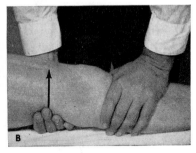

FIGURE 78A. The manner in which the anterior phase of the anteroposterior glide is performed when the knee is in fixed extension. Note the examiner's right hand stabilizes the femoral condyles, and his left hand mobilizes (in direction of arrow) the tibial condyles upon them.

FIGURE 78B. The manner in which the posterior phase of the anteroposterior glide is performed when the knee is in fixed extension. Note the examiner's left hand stabilizes the tibial condyles, and his right hand lifts (in direction of arrow) the femoral condyles upon them.

mal with the knee in midflexion. It is possible to produce a minimal degree of anteroposterior glide with the leg in extension. The anterior phase is performed by lifting the tibial condyles upward from the examining couch, while the femoral condyles are being held down on the couch (Figure 78A). The posterior phase of the movement is elicited by lifting the femoral condyles upward, while the tibial condyles are maintained on the examining couch (Figure 78B).

Rotation. To elicit the joint-play movement of rotation of the tibial condyles on the stabilized femoral condyles, the examiner grasps the thigh anteriorly over the femoral condyles with

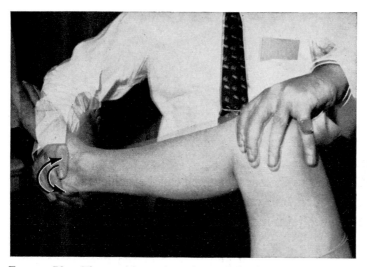

FIGURE 79. The position adopted to elicit the joint-play movement of rotation of the tibial condyles upon the femoral condyles (right knee). The double exposure illustrates the amount of rotation that is possible. The examiner's left hand stabilizes the femoral condyles, and his right hand rotates the tibia in its long axis through his grasp upon the calcaneus. The extent of the movement varies with the angle of flexion or extension of the knee; maximal rotation occurs with the knee in midflexion.

one hand, and with the other grasps the calcaneus on either side from beneath the heel, keeping his forearm in line with the lower leg. Then, he alternately supinates and pronates his forearm, rotating the tibial condyles clockwise and counterclockwise. Figure 79 shows the position adopted to elicit maximal joint-play rotation with the knee in midflexion, and the double exposure is made at the extremes of rotation, indicating the normal range.

Maximal rotation occurs at midflexion and decreases in extent as full extension or flexion is achieved. There is no rotation of the tibial condyles with the knee in full extension because of the "screw-to" locking mechanism of the quadriceps. Rotation elicited in full extension means impairment of quadriceps function.

The Patellofemoral Joint

The joint-play movements at this joint consist of an excursion of the patella cephalad, caudad, medially, and laterally independently of quadriceps movement and with the knee stabilized in extension.

Only the cephalad excursion can be achieved by voluntary muscle action, the other movements being purely involuntary. But no knee joint movement can take place if these involuntary movements are lost. In all the pathological conditions that affect the knee joint, atrophy and fibrosis of the quadriceps tend to pull the patella upward, where it tends to become fixed. If any therapeutic attempt is made to increase voluntary movement without first mobilizing the patella, it must fail and, indeed, there is danger, if the attempts are made forcefully, of fracturing the patella.

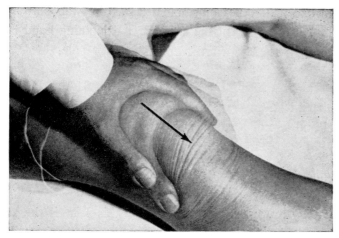

FIGURE 80. The position adopted to move the right patella down-ward (caudad). The thrust is entirely through the web between the examiner's thumb and index finger. The double exposure indicates the extent of this movement.

Caudad and Cephalad Excursions. Figure 80 shows how the thenar web is used to elicit the caudad joint-play movement of the patella. The double exposure indicates the wide range of normal movement. The cephalad movement of the patella is

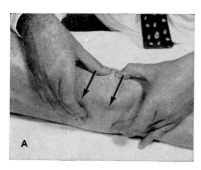

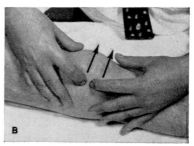

FIGURE 81A. The position adopted to elicit the medial range of the joint-play movement of the patella, the exposure being made at the medial limit of movement.

FIGURE 81B. The position adopted to elicit the lateral range of the joint-play movement of the patella, the exposure being made at the lateral limit of movement.

elicited in exactly the same manner but the web between the thumb and forefinger of the examiner's examining hand is used to push the patella upward from its inferior pole.

Lateral and Medial Excursions. Figures 81A and 81B show how the index fingers and the thumbs are used to elicit the medial and lateral joint-play movements of the patella.

The Superior Tibiofibular Joint

The only movement of joint play at this joint is the antero-posterior glide. The range of this movement varies with the degree of knee flexion and is absent with the knee in full exten-

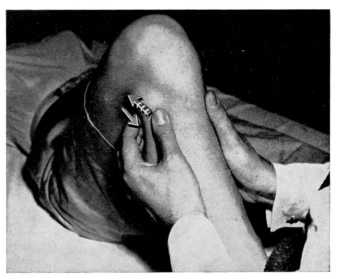

FIGURE 82. The position adopted to elicit the anteroposterior movement at the right superior tibiofibular joint. The exposure is made at the limit of the anterior phase of the movement. The examiner's right hand stabilizes the tibia, while his left hand mobilizes the head of the fibula.

sion. It is maximal with the knee in midflexion and is most easily demonstrated in this position.

The examiner sits on the subject's foot with the knee in the required angle of flexion. The head of the fibula is grasped between the thumb anteriorly and the tips of the index and middle fingers posteriorly, and the fingers and thumb then push forward and backward alternately. Figure 82 shows the examining position at the completion of the anterior phase of the movement.

13

The Hip

The hip joint is probably the most nearly perfect joint in the body. It is close to being a perfect ball-and-socket joint. There is only one movement of joint play at the hip, namely, long axis extension.

Long Axis Extension. To elicit this movement of joint play, the subject lies in the recumbent supine position, the weight of his body stabilizing the acetabulum. The head of the femur is then pulled away from the acetabulum in the long axis. To achieve this, the examiner grasps at arm's length the subject's lower leg around the ankle, and positions the leg in its neutral

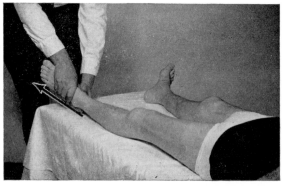

FIGURE 83.   The position adopted to elicit the joint-play movement of long axis extension at the hip.

rest position in a few degrees of abduction and external rotation. The examiner then exerts a pull downward in the long axis of the leg. The position adopted to elicit this movement is shown in Figure 83.

Loss of Extension. When there is dysfunction in the hip, it usually presents as limitation of extension of the joint. This seldom, if ever, happens unless there are pre-existing changes within the joint such as one sees with osteoarthritis. It is quite a common experience to see a patient with pain in the hip joint and with some loss of extension but remarkably full of flexion, who on radiographic examination appears to have practically no joint space in the hip joint. One wonders how there can be any movement at all in such a joint. It is my experience that restoration of the lost movement of extension does relieve symptoms of pain in these osteoarthritic joints. If a direct attempt is made forcefully to extend such a joint, there is a very definite danger of producing a torsion fracture in the neck of the femur.

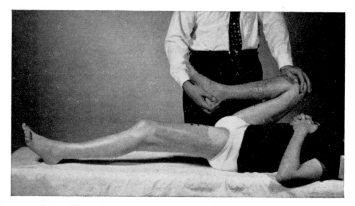

FIGURE 84. The classic examining position for loss of extension in an osteoarthritic hip joint. In this case the affected left hip with its loss of extension results in the left leg being raised off the couch before the right leg is fully flexed.

Therapeutically, however, it is possible to rotate the pelvis on the head of the femur when the joint changes are unilateral, which, fortunately, most often is the case. The left hip is used to illustrate this maneuver.

The loss of extension in a hip joint in cases of unilateral disease is commonly demonstrated by flexing the hip and the knee on the contralateral side and noting that the thigh of the affected leg rises from the couch before the unaffected leg is fully flexed (Figure 84).

Method of Restoring Lost Extension. To increase extension in the affected joint by rotating the pelvis upon the head of the affected femur, this clinical test maneuver is utilized. First, the good hip is fully flexed and, of course, the thigh on the affected side rises from the couch. Now the degree of flexion on the right unaffected side is released to the point at which the thigh of the left affected side is again flat upon the couch. At this

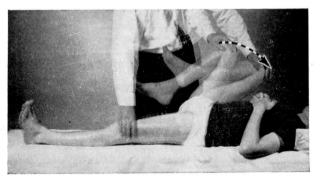

FIGURE 85. The method by which extension is restored to the left hip joint by rotating the pelvis upon the head of the affected femur. The examiner's right hand stabilizes the knee of the model's affected leg flat against the couch, while his left hand increases the flexion on the unaffected side. The double exposure, when it is compared with Figure 84, shows the wide movement that has to be used to produce not more than 10 degrees of additional extension.

point the examiner holds the left knee down by pressing with his right hand over the femoral condyles. With his left hand he increases the flexion of the right hip. In this way the pelvis rotates forward on the immobile head of the left femur producing extension in the left hip joint. The extent of the manipulative movement is shown by double exposure in Figure 85. This maneuver should be performed only after the joint-play movement of long axis extension in the affected hip has been restored.

14

Therapeutic Manipulation

Rules of Manipulation

Just as there are rules of technique to be followed when examining a joint, so there are rules of technique when manipulation is used to restore lost or impaired movements of joint play to normal. For the most part, the rules of technique for examination and for manipulation are the same, just as the movements used in therapy are, for the most part, the same as those used in examination. These rules, now modified for therapy, are of sufficient importance to reiterate them as follows:

1. The patient must be relaxed, and each aspect of the joint being treated must be supported and protected from unguarded, painful movement that may otherwise occur in the course of the premanipulative positioning.

2. The therapist must be relaxed. At no time must his therapeutic grasp be painful to the patient. It must be firm and protective, not gripping and restrictive.

3. One joint must be mobilized at a time. For instance, the wrist is not manipulated but the radiocarpal joint, the midcarpal joint, the ulnomeniscocarpal joint, and then the inferior radio-ulnar joint are each moved in turn.

4. One movement at each joint is restored at a time.

5. In the performance of any one movement, one facet of

the joint being mobilized is moved upon the other facet of the joint, which is stabilized. Thus, there should always be one mobilizing force and one stabilizing force exerted when a joint is being moved.

6. The extent of normal joint play can usually be assessed by examining the same joint on the opposite, unaffected limb, and the mobilizing force must never carry the joint being mobilized beyond this extent.

7. No forceful or abnormal movement must ever be used.

8. The manipulative movement used is a sharp springing thrust, push or pull, and must be differentiated from a forceful movement, which denotes lack of control of it. An uncontrolled movement is an abnormal movement. No therapeutic movement used while a patient is unconscious should have any more force behind it than would be used if the patient were conscious.

9. The springing movement is imparted to the joint only after taking up the slack in the joint to the point of pain. Then the movement is taken through this pain point to the limit of normal movement. A mobilizing movement starts at, and goes through, the point at which pain is elicited and at which the examination is stopped.

10. In the presence of clinical signs of joint or bone inflammation or disease, no therapeutic movements need be or should be undertaken.

Fractional Manipulation

In the large joints, for example, the shoulder, hip, and knee, the use of fractional manipulative techniques often must be used. Fractional manipulation means just going through each pain point and stopping without attempting to restore the full range of each movement at one session. Any gains in voluntary function resulting from the first session are maintained and consolidated by muscle re-education before the next session of mobilization is undertaken. Often the gain achieved by one fractional mobilization session is so improved on by the after-treatment that further sessions to increase the range of movement are unnecessary.

Use of Anesthesia in Manipulation

For some reason, controversy always arises when the subject of joint manipulation under anesthesia is brought up. It is perfectly safe to manipulate a joint with a patient anesthetized providing no departure is made from the specific normal manipulative techniques described. Certainly it is dangerous to manipulate a joint with the aid of anesthesia if the manipulator does anything more by force to a joint than he would were his patient conscious, or if he moves the joint in an abnormal way. Anesthesia is used only to obtain perfect control over a joint by eliminating resistive muscle spasm which cannot be eliminated by other means. It is used to spare the patient pain. It is used to prevent the use of force, not to facilitate it.

Local Anesthesia. In practice, I have found that few shoulder manipulations can be satisfactorily performed without the aid of anesthesia. For some reason, therapeutic manipulation of the glenohumeral joint is often very painful during its performance, but if the techniques that I have advocated are used, there is practically no after-pain.

I have recently used brachial plexus blocks to provide shoulder joint anesthesia when performing therapeutic manipulation of this joint. It is useful if a patient is a poor risk for general anesthesia. It has, however, two drawbacks: first, the patient cannot move the joint through its voluntary range until the block wears off, which may take some hours; and second, the patient experiences considerable psychological trauma when he hears the noise accompanying the manipulative movements, feeling, at the same time, the arm to be "dead." When pentothal is used for general anesthesia, the patient is able to move his arm through its restored range, certainly within thirty minutes, and thus can maintain the increased range attained. With the brachial plexus block, the joint tends to stiffen up again in the hours required for recovery of muscle action.

Intra-articular Injection. Local anesthesia instilled into the smaller joints often relieves pain sufficiently to produce adequate relaxation to allow them to be manipulated. In some of the larger joints, but particularly the hip and the knee, I use a "lactocaine" solution injected intra-articularly. The solution is made up freshly, using the following prescription: lactic acid, 0.2 per cent, is combined with procaine, 1 per cent, and the solution is buffered to a pH of 5.2 and sterilized. About 8 cc. of the solution is injected into these joints. One supposes that the bulk of fluid injected tends to stretch the capsule of the joint, which in these cases may be fibrotic and adherent. One also supposes that the fluid cushions the articulating surfaces of the joint while the local anesthetic temporarily relieves the capsular pain. So, when the capsule is stretched during the manipulation, pain from it does not produce reflex muscle spasm to resist the movement.

I cannot see that it is any more or less rational or safe to use anesthesia to avoid pain during joint manipulation intended to restore normal movement and to achieve freedom from pain than it is to use it during the reduction of fractures and dislocations or, for that matter, during extraction of a tooth.

15

Special Therapeutic Techniques

The Fingers

The reader will remember that in the section dealing with examination of the fingers, attention was drawn to the radial relationship of the articular surfaces of the head of the metacarpal bone and the base of the proximal phalanx, which remains constant at rest and in voluntary movement (Figure 86A). (See also Figures 2, 4, and 10 on pages 33, 34, and 37.) Clearly, this illustrates that the movements of the metacarpophalangeal joints (and the interphalangeal joints) bear no true relationship to the movements of a hinge.

When restoring movement to these joints therapeutically — particularly the movements of flexion and extension — if the therapist simply tries to bend the joint forward or backward as he might a hinge, he may, by force, alter the radial relationship of the articular surfaces of the bones he is moving, and this is abnormal. If he persists, he will either fracture the anterior or posterior lip of the base of the phalanx (depending on whether he is trying to force flexion or extension), or he will rupture the collateral ligaments by stretching them abnormally, as the radius of the arc of the circle around which their phalangeal attachment moves is being forcibly lengthened. Figures 86A and 86B diagrammatically illustrate what must happen if a forceful attempt is made to flex the joint, disregarding the fact that in

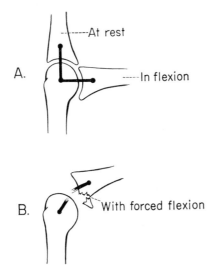

FIGURE 86. (A) Diagrammatic illustration of the lateral view of a metacarpophalangeal joint at rest and in flexion. The constant radial relationship of the base of the phalanx should be noted. (B) Illustration of what must happen if any attempt at forced flexion of a metacarpophalangeal joint is made with any amount of leverage and if the joint is treated as a hinge.

normal voluntary movement the articular surfaces maintain their same radial relationship throughout movement.

Therapeutic Maneuver to Restore Flexion. To restore manipulatively the normal movements in the range of joint play in the finger joints is not sufficient when attempting to increase the voluntary range of these joints. After restoring the joint-play movements, it is still necessary to try to reproduce the normal gliding motion of the base of the phalanx around the head of the metacarpal bone (or the base of a more distal phalanx around the phalanx immediately proximal to it); this demands the use of a special technique if the base of the phalanx being moved is to remain undamaged and the collateral ligaments are to remain inviolate.

Using the metacarpophalangeal joint of the index finger of

the left hand for illustration, let us first suppose that it is fixed in extension. The examiner places the thumb of his left hand just proximal to the head of the metacarpal bone on its palmar aspect with his terminal thumb phalanx at right angles to the shaft of the subject's metacarpal bone. The examiner places the thumb of his right hand just distal to the base of the proximal phalanx of the subject's index finger on its dorsal aspect, his terminal thumb phalanx being at right angles to the shaft of the subject's phalanx. The examiner stabilizes the head of the metacarpal bone with his left thumb and pushes the base of the subject's proximal phalanx around the head of the metacarpal bone with his right thumb, the thrust being kept at a right angle throughout the movement. The radial relationship of the articulating surfaces of the bones is thus maintained at all times.

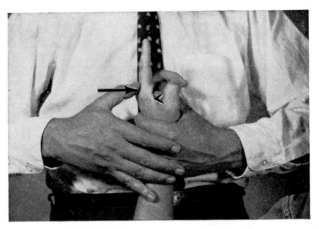

FIGURE 87. The position adopted to reproduce the movement of true flexion at a stiff metacarpophalangeal joint. The examiner's left thumb stabilizes the head of the model's metacarpal bone on its palmar surface, while his right thumb pushes the base of the model's phalanx around it. Arrow shows direction of thrust, whereas wedge indicates point of stabilization.

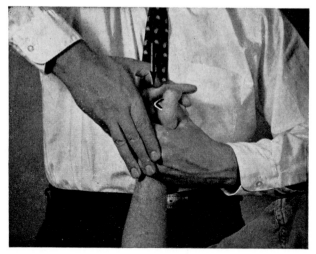

FIGURE 88.   The position of the examiner's thumbs at the completion of the flexion movement, the start of which is shown in Figure
87. Note that the terminal phalanx of the mobilizing thumb remains
at right angles to the model's proximal phalanx, just as it was at the
beginning of the movement.

Figure 87 illustrates the position adopted at the beginning
of this movement; Figure 88 illustrates the position at the end
of the movement. It should be noted that the position of the
examiner's left thumb is not altered, whereas his right thumb
at the beginning of the movement is parallel to the left one and
at the end of the movement is at right angles to it.

Therapeutic Maneuver to Restore Extension. If the subject's finger is stiff in the flexed position, the role of the examiner's thumbs is exactly reversed. The examiner now places his
left thumb just distal to the base of the subject's proximal phalanx on its palmar aspect and thrusts the base of the phalanx
around the head of the metacarpal bone until extension is
achieved. Meanwhile the examiner's right thumb stabilizes the
head of the metacarpal bone on its dorsal aspect. Figure 89

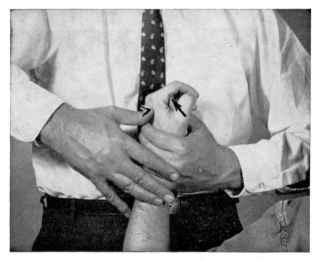

FIGURE 89. The position adopted to reproduce the movement of
true extension at a metacarpophalangeal joint fixed in flexion. The
examiner's right thumb stabilizes the head of the metacarpal bone
on its dorsal surface, while his left thumb pushes the base of the
phalanx around it.

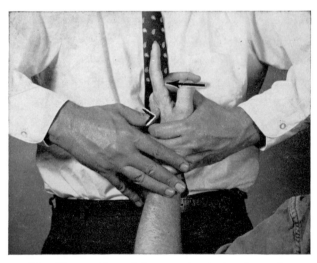

FIGURE 90. The position of the examiner's thumbs at the completion of the movement of extension at a metacarpophalangeal joint.

shows the position adopted at the beginning of the movement, when it will be noted that the examiner's thumbs are at right angles to each other. The position at the end of the movement is shown in Figure 90, the examiner's thumbs having now arrived in a position in which they are parallel to each other.

The Elbow

There is a clinical condition at the elbow which simulates a meniscus derangement at the radiohumeral joint, but is postulated as being due to an adherent scar following a tear of the fibers of the common extensor tendon close to its origin at the lateral condyle of the humerus. The chief clinical feature that distinguishes this from a meniscus injury is the accurate location of pain on palpation. With the latter the maximum pain on palpation lies over the head of the radius, whereas the maximum pain on palpation of the soft tissue injury is proximal to and more lateral than the radial head. The close relationship of these two anatomical points is shown in Figure 91.

Differential Diagnosis of Pain from Meniscus Injury and from Soft Tissue Scar. In addition, there is a very reliable electrical test that is positive when the pathological condition is in the tendon, but is negative when the injury is in the joint. The area of palpation that is tender when there is a scar in the tendon is very localized and can be easily found by applying pressure with the eraser end of a pencil; it is usually no larger than this. If one marks the tender area, and then with a button

---

Note that the terminal phalanx of the mobilizing thumb remains at right angles to the model's proximal phalanx, as it was at the beginning of the movement (see Figure 89).

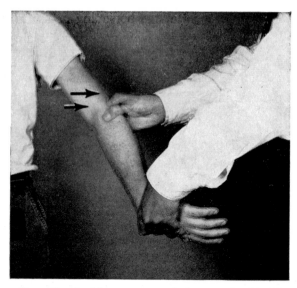

FIGURE 91. The double exposure of the examiner's right thumb shows the close relationship between the area where pain is elicited due to dysfunction at the superior radioulnar joint (lower arrow) and where pain is elicited when there is a tear in the common extensor tendon (upper arrow).

electrode conveying a faradic current strokes around the area, using a subtonal current, the patient will experience pain under the electrode in exactly the same place where he experienced pain on palpation.

Therapeutic Maneuver to Tear Painful Scar in Common Extensor Tendon. The treatment for a painful scar in the common extensor tendon is to tear the scar and then to treat it as a recent injury should be treated. The tearing of the scar can be achieved by using the following manipulative technique, the left elbow being used for illustration.

The examiner grasps the patient's upper arm over the posterior aspect of the humerus at the elbow with his right hand, the thumb resting over the area of the tendon which is painful on palpation. With his left hand, he grasps the subject's wrist over its posterior aspect and then flexes the elbow fully, pronates the forearm fully, and flexes the wrist fully. The examiner now extends the patient's elbow. As the extensor muscles tighten toward the end of this extension movement (maintaining full pronation of the forearm and full flexion of the wrist at all times), the examiner feels resistance to the movement, and the patient experiences pain under the examiner's right thumb. The examiner then whips the elbow into full extension, at which moment the patient experiences an acute transitory pain as the scar tears. This procedure is more comfortable if the tender area is first infiltrated with a local anesthetic. Figure 92 illus-

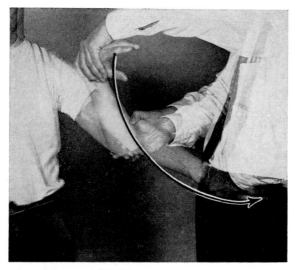

FIGURE 92. The position adopted to perform the therapeutic movement of manipulation by which the common extensor tendon is put on stretch to tear a scar in it. It should be noted that the forearm is in full pronation and the wrist in full flexion, these positions being maintained throughout the movement. The position at the end of this movement is also shown in Figure 91. Line of arrow shows path of examiner's left (mobilizing) hand during movement.

trates the position adopted to perform this movement, and the double exposure illustrates the extent of the movement.

The Shoulder

When restoring the movements of joint play to a shoulder in which there is dysfunction, the sequence in which the movements are restored follows the same sequence as that described in the examination procedures in Chapter 8, pages 78–86. Before this sequence of therapeutic techniques is started, however, an additional therapeutic maneuver of long axis extension should be done. The head of the humerus is pulled away from the glenoid cavity in the long axis of the arm with the arm at the maximum angle of abduction that is possible for the patient without pain. This angle of abduction may vary from almost zero degrees to approximately 120 degrees, at which point all the big muscles of the shoulder girdle are pulling from the chest wall into the arm in an almost perfect conelike manner. Indeed, if the technique of fractional manipulation is being employed, full painless movement of the shoulder may not be achieved until long axis extension at this 120-degree angle is carried out. The performance of this movement may be the final therapeutic maneuver necessary to bring success to the treatment being undertaken. In the following description of this maneuver, the left arm is used for illustrative purposes.

Long Axis Extension at the Glenohumeral Joint. Figure 93 illustrates the most convenient method of performing long axis extension with the arm at its maximum angle of abduction. The examiner's foot stabilizes the scapula, that is, the glenoid cavity, and the head of the humerus is pulled away from it by a pull

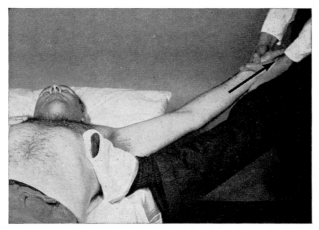

FIGURE 93.   The method of long axis extension at the glenohumeral joint with the arm in full abduction. Arrow shows direction
of pull.

exerted from the patient's wrist. Figures 94A and 94B show the
same maneuver being performed with the patient's arm at a
minimal angle of abduction, and in this instance the glenoid

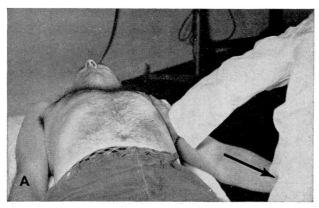

FIGURE 94A.   The method adopted to perform long axis extension at the glenohumeral joint when only minimal abduction of the
patient's arm is possible. Arrow indicates direction of mobilizing
pull by examiner's right hand.

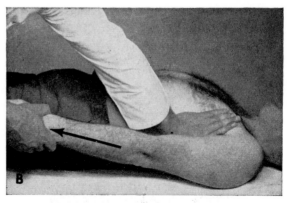

FIGURE 94B.   Side view of the position adopted to perform long axis extension at the glenohumeral joint when only minimal abduction of the patient's arm is possible. Note that the arm must not be forward flexed, but that it is raised from the couch to counteract the amount of extension that occurs normally when one lies down.

cavity is stabilized by pressure of the examiner's left hand in the axilla, and the head of the humerus is mobilized by a pull of the examiner's right hand grasping the left wrist of the patient.

When the cause of the patient's shoulder disability appears on examination to be chiefly due to a loss of that movement of joint play in which the head of his humerus is pulled downward and backward within the glenoid cavity (as described in the examining maneuvers in Chap. 8, page 82), there is a reasonably facile manner in which this can be restored with the patient standing. The examiner stands with his back to the patient, who places his left side next to the examiner's back and faces away from the examiner's left side toward his right side. The examiner then drapes the patient's arm over his left shoulder and clasps the upper arm over the surgical neck of the humerus. The patient is inclined over the examiner's back in such a manner that his arm is hanging vertically toward the floor. The examiner's knees are bent. The position adopted in

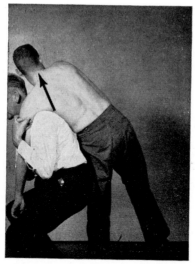

FIGURE 95. The position adopted to perform a therapeutic maneuver for pulling the head of the humerus downward within the glenoid cavity. Note that the examiner is grasping the model's arm around the surgical neck of the humerus and that the pull is directly toward the floor. In performing the maneuver the arm remains stabilized and the glenoid cavity is pushed upward upon the head of the humerus by a thrust through the examiner's shawl area. Figure 96 shows the wrong and dangerous way of performing the maneuver.

performing this therapeutic maneuver correctly is shown in Figure 95. As the examiner extends his knees, he stabilizes the upper end of the patient's humerus over his clavicle. As the patient is lifted from the floor slightly, the glenoid cavity (scapula) moves upward on the head of the humerus, which, in fact, means that the head of the humerus is moving downward and backward within the glenoid cavity. There is danger to this movement if the examiner's shoulder is being used as a fulcrum under the surgical neck of the patient's humerus and if the examiner grasps the patient's forearm too close to the elbow. A fracture can easily result through the neck of the patient's humerus because of the forces of leverage being exerted. Figure 96 illus-

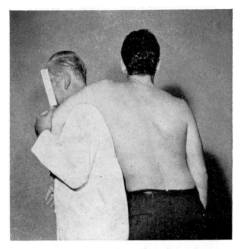

FIGURE 96. The wrong way of performing the therapeutic maneuver to pull the head of the humerus downward within the glenoid cavity, and this figure should be compared with Figure 95. In this illustration the examiner's shawl area is being used as a fulcrum and the model's upper arm as a lever. A fracture through the surgical neck of the humerus could easily result when the examiner exerts the therapeutic lift.

trates the incorrect position, so easily adopted, in performing this maneuver.

The Knee

Therapeutic Maneuver to Increase Range of Flexion at Knee. The reader will remember that, when the restoration of flexion to a finger was being discussed, attention was drawn to the fact that the articular surfaces of the metacarpal bone and the phalanx glided around each other and acted in no way like a hinge. The same thing holds for flexion and extension of the knee joint. Here again, the tibial condyle glides around the condyles of the femur in the arc of the circle whose center is the attachment of the collateral ligaments of the femoral condyles and whose radius is the length of the collateral ligaments. So, in a knee that is fixed in extension, it is not always sufficient to restore the movements of joint play when a therapeutic attempt is being made to restore flexion to the joint. There is an additional therapeutic manipulative maneuver that may be applied, but only when the technique of fractional manipulation is being used. This technique must never be used until the full range of joint-play movements of the patella is restored and the other movements of joint play between the femoral condyles and tibial condyles have been restored. Having restored all these movements in the range of joint play, the following additional flexion technique may be applied, with caution. The left knee is used for illustration.

The subject lies supine on the couch and the examiner stands or sits at his left side. The examiner abducts the subject's leg sufficiently so that the knee and lower leg are over the edge of the couch. The examiner then places his right forearm in the popliteal area, resting the posterior aspect of the subject's tibial condyles upon it, and grasps the subject's ankle over its anterior aspect with his left hand. While pulling the tibial condyles forward with his right forearm, the examiner exerts a flexion pressure at the knee by thrusting with his left hand at the subject's ankle. Figure 97 illustrates the position adopted for the performance of this maneuver. The manipulative thrust must stop as soon as the lower leg moves through its first dead point, that is, as soon as something "gives" in the knee.

Therapeutic Maneuver to Overcome a Medial Meniscus Block. A patient's knee may lock in flexion due to internal derangement of the medial meniscus without the meniscus being torn. When this happens, the normal anatomical functional position of the meniscus and normal function of the knee can be

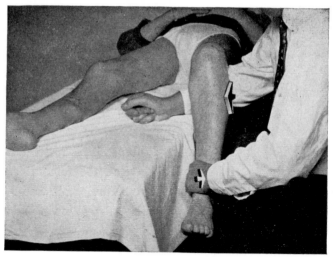

FIGURE 97. The position adopted to increase the range of flexion
at the knee. For the most part, the tibial condyles are pulled forward by the examiner's right forearm as the primary mobilizing
force, while his left hand carries the leg through the small arc of
movement achieved.

restored by the following manipulative technique. The left knee
is used for illustration.

The examiner stands on the left of the subject and grasps the
calcaneus on its plantar aspect with his left hand. The examiner
places the palm of his right hand over the lateral aspect of the
knee joint and carries the subject's knee into full flexion, which
means, of course, that the hip is also carried into full flexion.
The examiner then externally rotates the tibial condyles through
the long axis of the tibia by turning the calcaneus clockwise.
It should be noted that in addition to the twist on the calcaneus,
the examiner's left forearm rests against the medial aspect of
the patient's foot, thereby giving additional control to this
mobilizing maneuver. At the same time, and to keep the leg
in the saggital plane, pressure is exerted by the examiner's
right hand medially against the lateral femoral condyle. If there

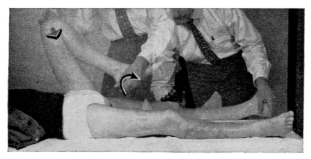

FIGURE 98. The starting position and the finishing position, by double exposure, of the therapeutic maneuver to free a locked knee because of a medial meniscus derangement. Note that the examiner's right hand maintains a thrust medially from the lateral surface of the knee and that his left hand maintains external rotation of the tibial condyles by its grasp on the calcaneus with the examiner's wrist resting along the medial aspect of the model's foot.

is a limitation of flexion, the examiner first carries the knee into full flexion and immediately whips it out into full extension. Figure 98 illustrates the starting and finishing positions of this maneuver. The secret to success in using this therapeutic maneuver is that the external rotation of the tibial condyles and the medial pressure through the examiner's right hand at the knee, which tends to open the medial aspect of the joint, are at no time relaxed during the performance of the extension movement. The double exposure attempts to show the extent of this movement.

16

Osteoarthritis and Joint Pain

Probably the commonest diagnosis for the cause of pain in the synovial joint used in clinical practice today is that of arthritis. Of course, this is a meaningless term unless there is a descriptive prefix attached to it and what is invariably meant in this connotation is osteoarthritis.

Diagnosis of Osteoarthritis

Radiographic Changes and Joint Pain. The diagnosis is based upon characteristic subchondral bone changes visualized on radiographic examination of a joint, without any real thought being given to what the pictorial changes may represent if related to the living function of the joint. The condition is often explained away to a patient as being due to unfair wear and tear, and the inference is implied, if not actually stated, that the changes are irreversible and that therefore the patient must expect to suffer from and with them.

If a patient comes into the office with a painful knee and gives a history that 2 or 3 weeks ago he twisted his knee, that it swelled and was painful, and that the pain is persisting longer than he would expect following simple strain of a joint, and if an x-ray is taken of this joint and radiographic changes char-

154

acteristic of osteoarthritis are revealed, then it is common practice to tell the patient that the cause of his pain is osteoarthritis. It is then usual to prescribe, rather empirically, heat, quadriceps-strengthening exercises, indefinite periods of rest, and maybe a weight-reducing diet. Some specific thing may be done to the joint itself, and fortunately it is not too uncommon that the patient is relieved of his pain, at least for a time. If another x-ray is now taken, there would, of course, be no change in the radiographic picture — the changes characteristic of osteoarthritis would still be there as large as life. Yet, for some reason, the symptom of pain has disappeared.

Cause of Pain in the Osteoarthritic Joint. There is, of course, no anatomical, physiological, or pathological reason why osteoarthritis should give rise to pain. If there were, it would be reasonable to tell a patient that not too much can be done to alleviate the symptoms other than relieving the joint of weight bearing, if it is in the lower limbs, or from use, if it is in the upper limbs. Certainly, there is a wearing away of the hyaline cartilage in an osteoarthritic joint, and when this is gross, it may be that bone might rub upon bone and give rise to pain symptoms. But so long as the articulating bony surface is covered by any cartilage at all, there is no reason why pain should arise from this simple wearing-away process since, of course, the hyaline cartilage does not have any nerve supply.

Since empirical treatment is often successful in alleviating pain in osteoarthritic joints, there must be, in its wide variety, a common denominator in which lies the key to the true nature of the cause of pain and, therefore, a more logical and sure way of treatment.

Perhaps the most interesting or, should one say, confusing treatment that often proves to be the most successful in relieving pain is that of intra-articular injection of some drug or chemical. Currently hydrocortisone, or one of the newer steroid preparations, is most commonly used. Acid potassium phosphate with procaine, or lactic acid with procaine, or air have been as commonly used. These substances have little in common with each other except the property of either analgesia or a cushioning effect, or both. The large amount of fluid used with lactic acid and acid potassium phosphate injection almost certainly stretches the joint capsule since, of course, fluid is incompressible and something has to give.

There is no very logical reason why any of these intra-articular injections, of themselves, should be permanently effective. It is my thesis that in those cases in which it is effective, Nature resolves some unrecognized impairment of the function of the joint through an accidental unguarded movement while the joint is thus made analgesic or is cushioned.

Abnormal Movement in the Osteoarthritic Joint. Associated with these characteristic osteoarthritic changes in the synovial joint is a loss of space-occupying mass between the articulating bones, and this allows for a slackening of the supporting ligaments or muscles, or both, of the joint. Because of this, abnormal movement of the joint may and does take place. Sooner or later there is an associated thickening of the capsule with loss of elasticity and increase of fibrosis. With increased fibrosis there is contraction. This means that the capsule of the joint tightens around it. This tightening of the capsule may compensate for some of the excess movement that is allowed by the loss of the cartilage space-occupying mass. Equally, it may overcompensate and prevent normal movement. When one uses the term "normal movement" in relation to joint function, one must remember that both types of movement are affected, that is, the normal voluntary and joint-play movements.

Manipulation in Treatment of the Osteoarthritic Joint

If osteoarthritic joints are examined, using the techniques that I have described, when pain is present, invariably one will find signs that are characteristic of joint dysfunction, which means a loss of one or more of the normal joint-play movements.

Osteoarthritis, except in its grossest forms is then a painless change which occurs in the synovial joints because of specific major or repetitive minor traumas to them. Pain in an osteoarthritic joint arises from a loss of one or more movements in the normal range of movement that is not under the control of voluntary-muscle action, and in this regard I postulate the existence of a specific range of movement at every synovial joint in the body that I have called the range of movement of joint play. Pain in these synovial joints can be relieved by the restoration of this lost movement by joint manipulation. I suggest that, when manipulation is not used, success in treatment for the relief of pain occurs only with the fortuitous intervention of Nature providing an accidental manipulative stress, while analgesia or cushioning is produced in the joint by other nonspecific methods of treatment or, if analgesia is not practiced, by unnecessary painful and traumatic treatment or accident. Such a joint may be kept symptom free by maintaining the integrity of its supporting musculature and by prophylactic attention to the mechanics of weight bearing, not only at the involved joint but in all related weight-bearing joints. In addition, attention to the amount of weight to be borne and a prescription of adequate rest must be given besides attention to and the correction of acquired postural anomalies.

Although this thesis may have its practical limitations, it emphasizes the importance of assessing the patient as a whole rather than dissecting him into parts, which is an unfortunate tendency in clinical practice.

Osteoarthritis too often is a poor excuse for a diagnosis of the cause of pain and an even poorer one for the prescription of empirical treatment since, even though the treatment for pain in an osteoarthritic joint may be successful, the osteoarthritic changes persist. These changes, therefore. can play little, if any, part in the production of symptoms until they are so gross that destruction of the joint by fusion offers the only chance of relieving the pain; it should be possible to prevent this end result.

It is my belief that osteoarthritic changes start because of the poor management of acute joint injury in early years. There are clear clinical indications in treating acutely traumatized joints that all is well again with the joint and that it is ready to resume its function. The chief signs that all is not well are the presence of an excess of synovial fluid within a joint — synovitis — and atrophy of any of the muscles acting upon the joint. If, following a traumatic incident, a patient is allowed to resume the use of that joint before the excess of synovial fluid is absorbed or before the atrophied muscle is restored to normal, it surely means that the traumatic effects of the injury are not healed. If the joint is then used, it is being abused, and it is only reasonable to expect changes of osteoarthritis to appear in it as the years go by.

Restoration of the lost movement of joint play relieves the symptom of pain if it is due to joint dysfunction. Normal movement to the painful joint having been restored and pain in it

having been relieved, recurrences can be prevented by prophylactic measures.

Prophylactic Treatment Against Joint Pain

Physical Therapy. Pain in a joint produces spasm of its
supporting muscles, and if spasm is prolonged, it will produce
atrophy in them. An integral part of prophylactic treatment, then,
is the development and re-education of the supporting musculature. The quickest and most efficient way to achieve this is
the prescription of exercise to the affected muscle, or muscles,
without function of the joint. This means, in the lower limb,
without weight bearing, or in the joints of the upper limb, without the strain of too early use. Too early return to use of a
recently painful joint without its being adequately supported
by its stabilizing and mobilizing musculature can only court an
early recurrence of joint dysfunction if the joint is subject to
further unguarded stress.

It is commonly said that such exercise treatment can be carried out by a patient without the supervision of a well-qualified
physical therapist. If the physician provides time to instruct
the patient specifically in the physiological and anatomical movement of muscle, and if the patient is intelligent and receptive
and is well motivated, this may well be true. My experience
is that these prerequisites to success of an exercise program are
in fact very rare.

The metronomic contraction and relaxation of muscle in no
way bears any relationship to the normal physiology of muscle
movement. Repetitive contraction and relaxation that ignores
the relaxation period and refractory period of muscle can only
produce fatigue in it, and this results in nonphysiological muscle

action that may well produce the exact opposite effect of re-training that the prescribed exercise program is designed to achieve. Each movement in exercise treatment must be properly performed to be of any use. The joint to be treated must be adequately supported to prevent the forces of gravity acting as a counterforce against muscle action. When function is first resumed as treatment progresses, the joint should be adequately supported if it is a weight-bearing joint. All exercise should be kept within the limit of pain. It must be stressed that no muscle can be re-educated and restored to normal if the joint which it moves is not free to move through its normal range of movement. In other words, restoration of joint movement is a prerequisite to the re-education of muscle, for freedom of muscle movement necessary to the development of muscle volume and power demands that the muscle be able to contract through its full range.

Weight Bearing, Posture, and Occupational Factors. The affected joint must also be protected from certain stresses of weight bearing that will otherwise accelerate the changes of normal wear and tear. Wear and tear denotes repetitive minor trauma, with the hip joints and the knee joints usually being involved most often. It should be a matter of some comment that the other weight-bearing joints — namely, those of the feet and ankles and those of the spine — are less frequently affected, although they carry just as heavy a load. This is surely because in the feet and back the load is better distributed — in the feet and ankles by the multiplicity of joints and in the spine by the additional shock-absorbing arrangement of the intervertebral discs and by the multiplicity of joints. It should be remembered that lipping of vertebral bodies, which is so often called osteoarthritis, has, in fact, nothing to do with this condition at all.

Osteoarthritis, being a change peculiar to synovial joints, can appear only in the interlaminar joints, the sacroiliac joints, and the costovertebral joints in the spine. The non-weight-bearing synovial joints of the upper limbs are affected by osteoarthritis but only following gross trauma, or in certain occupations in which they are subjected to unusual repetitive trauma because of the nature of the work performed.

Joints are designed so that there is an optimum position in which the ill effects of weight bearing are minimal. (Normal posture with normal weight bearing in the weight-bearing joints is shown in Figure 99A.) Any deviation from this position encourages articular changes, because wear and tear is greater if the weight is borne by a part of the articular cartilage that was not designed to bear it.

Civilization, with its customs and diseases, has made it commonplace for human beings to lose at an early age the elasticity of their Achilles tendons. This frequently results in what we call an insufficiency of these tendons, which is evident to a greater or lesser degree by observing the position that the foot adopts at rest. When there is an insufficiency of the tendo-Achillis and a concomitant loss of resilience of muscle because of the natural aging process, or because of enforced disuse at a younger age, an undue stretch is put on the calf muscles if the os calcis is to reach the ground before or at the same time as the heads of the metartarsal bones, as in walking or standing (Figure 99B). In an attempt to compensate for this, there is an attempt to hyperextend the knee joints that results in an unnatural, constant backward bracing of them. The knee joints were not designed to bear weight constantly with their articular cartilages in contact in the braced position of the knee. Because of a loss of resilience in the thigh muscles and hip flexor muscles, there is now a tendency for the hip joint to be held in a position of partial

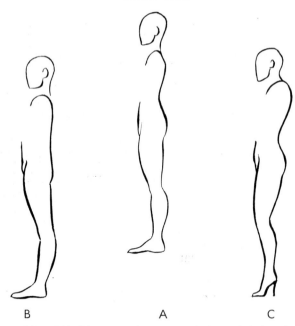

B   A   C

FIGURE 99.   (A) The normal posture of the weight-bearing joints
of the lower extremities and normal spinal curves with normally
resilient Achilles tendons. (B) The effect of tendo-Achillis insufficiency — extension of the knees and hips, flattening of the normal
spinal curves, and flattening of the arches in the feet. (C) The effect of wearing shoes with too high heels — flexion of the knees
and hips, accentuation of all of the spinal curves, and exaggeration
of the arches of the feet with abnormal weight bearing on the metatarsal heads.

extension. An unnatural weight-bearing aspect of the articular
cartilages of the femoral head and of the acetabulum is then subjected to undue stress. In an attempt to compensate for this, the
normal lumbar lordosis tends to become flattened, a condition
which in turn produces an unnatural postural strain on the
synovial interlaminar joints of the lumbar spine.

Frequently, the iliotibial bands also lose their elasticity, and
in becoming short and taut they prevent the normal gliding movement of the greater trochanters of the femora beneath them.

Instead, the greater trochanters carry the bands forward with them when one is walking, thereby instituting a constant rocking of the pelvis at the lumbosacral junction and an unnatural forward and backward torsion movement between the ilia and sacrum at the sacroiliac joints, not only producing traumatic osteoarthritic changes in these joints but, by stretching of their ligaments, making the joints at the lumbosacral junction more prone to lock and the sacroiliac joints more prone to subluxation. It is likely, too, that the resulting abnormal stresses on the fourth and fifth lumbar discs resulting from such excess movement may well be sufficient to initiate disc degeneration, or even a frank prolapse.

These postural errors of weight bearing produce stresses and strains such as those which a normal person experiences temporarily when he stands facing an incline, that is, when walking straight up a hill. Apart from the abnormal weight bearing so induced, it is noteworthy that the strain on the calf muscles under these circumstances, which prevents adequate relaxation of them, will sufficiently interfere with the circulation through them to produce the disabling symptoms of pseudo-intermittent claudication, a condition too often misdiagnosed as true intermittent claudication. The pain of the former condition is easily remedied by raising the heels of the patient's shoes.

In women who are accustomed to wearing shoes with too high heels, the reverse stresses at the joints that we have been discussing occur; the knees tend to be constantly flexed, the hips are constantly flexed, and the lumbar lordosis becomes exaggerated (Figure 99C). In these cases there is a greater tendency for the involvement of the joints of the thoracic and cervical spines as well, because of an increase in the thoracic kyphosis and the cervical lordosis by compensating mechanisms.

Thus, it will be seen that the prophylactic management of

osteoarthritis from a musculoskeletal postural point of view starts with the feet and footwear of the patient and works upward. There is a simple and expeditious method of determining the height which the heels of shoes should be to compensate for Achilles tendon insufficiency. A Duralumin strip is shaped to the contour of the inner border of the foot at rest (Figure 100).

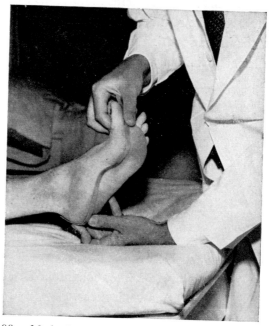

FIGURE 100. Method used to assess the contour of the foot at rest, the prerequisite of determining the heel height required to compensate for tendo-Achillis insufficiency.

This contoured strip is then removed from the foot and put on a firm table. A book is placed under the heel part of the metal strip and leafed open until the flat heel part of the strip is parallel to the floor (Figure 101). This height is measured and is the height of shoe heel required to correct the weight bearing of the weight-

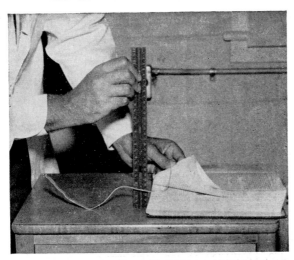

FIGURE 101. The duralumin strip is removed from the foot and the heel part of the contour is supported on an open book. The correct heel height is measured when the flat part of the heel contour is parallel to the table top.

bearing joints of the lower limb and spine. This height is by no means always the same on both sides.

However, full compensation is not recommended lest the remaining resilience in the tendons be lost. Also it must be remembered that ready-made store shoes can only have a maximum of ½ inch added to their heels without producing foot symptoms from too great an alteration of the slope of the soles of the shoes. Further, any addition of heel height to a ready-made shoe must be wedge-shaped and not just a block. If a block heel is added, the front of it will catch, and the shank will have to be broken down to allow the forepart of the shoe to contact the ground at the same time as the heel in standing. So, in practice, the maximum correction of the heel of a ready-made shoe is the addition of a heel wedge measuring ½ inch posteriorly, sloping forward to ¼ inch anteriorly. This gives a central heel lift of about ⅜ inch.

Other Prophylactic Factors. Having relieved the pain in an osteoarthritic joint, having re-educated and strengthened the supporting muscles of the involved joint, and having attempted to correct the postural stresses on the involved joint to the best of one's ability, there still remain four problems of management of the patient which are just as important as anything else — body weight, infections, occupational hazards, and rest.

The first problem, usually the most obvious one, is the maintenance of the body weight to that which the damaged joints may be expected to bear without further undue wear and tear. In this respect I believe that there is some relation in water balance to osteoarthritis, although I am not prepared to speculate on its nature. However, it has been my experience that patients who suffer from persistently painful osteoarthritic joints invariably are deficient in their daily fluid intake.

Second, the patient must attempt to avoid the development of any focus of infection which may become the cause of a low-grade infective arthritis in the osteoarthritic joint. Any focus of infection must be eradicated. While accepting that there are two schools of thought in regard to the part played by focal infection in the symptoms of osteoarthritis, it is my experience that symptoms persist in the presence of a focus of infection until it is eradicated.

Third, the patient should be removed from a causative occupational hazard, and, if necessary, vocational rehabilitation should be instituted. There are remarkable facilities available in this country about which too little is known even by some of the agencies that are set up to deal with these problems.

The fourth problem that confronts us in the management of the patient is to persuade him to rest sufficiently his already damaged joint each and every day and yet to maintain the integrity of his muscles.

17

Concepts and Conclusions

The concept of joint play as a prerequisite of normal voluntary joint movement is new. To many practitioners joint dysfunction, or the loss of movement in the range of joint play, as a cause of joint pain must remain hypothetical unless steps are taken to put the theory into practice. One thing that should make this theory attractive is that it is the only theory of a cause of pain that holds for every synovial joint wherever it may be in the body, without exception. Other schools of thought have one explanation for synovial joint pain in the weight-bearing joints of the lower extremities, another for it in the joints of the upper extremities, and yet others for pain in each section of the vertebral column.

The concept of intrinsic trauma as opposed to extrinsic trauma as a prerequisite of symptoms may also be new to some. The understanding that an unguarded movement superimposed on a joint that is going through a normal voluntary movement without stress can and does produce painful dysfunction is something which must be appreciated before anyone can look at manipulative techniques in diagnosis and treatment with an open mind.

At my annual post-graduate course on Joint Manipulation at the White Memorial Hospital in Los Angeles, my students are often initially impatient because I insist on spending so much

time on the first day demonstrating joint play at the metacarpophalangeal joint of an index finger and then on the other digital
joints. Yet, if the student cannot perfectly handle this, the simplest
joint in the body, he cannot be expected to handle the joints of
the spine, which can only be moved indirectly.

Further, it is basic to my thesis not only that each movement
of joint play at each joint should be elicited, but also that the loss
of one of these movements should be recognized and the cause
for its loss be determined. If it is lost as a part of — or a sign of
— any pathological condition in the joint other than simple
dysfunction, then any manipulative maneuvers imparted to the
joint can only be expected to aggravate the patient's symptoms
and their cause.

Thus in learning examining manipulative techniques, it is
necessary to learn them on normal joints. If the performance of
an examining movement causes any pain whatever in a normal
joint, then the movement is being performed incorrectly. If a
damaged joint is moved incorrectly, further damage is surely inflicted on it.

In teaching the subject, therefore, I pair off the students. I
demonstrate each normal movement to them, and then each student performs the same movement on his partner and has each
movement performed by his partner on him. I have found that
getting the feel of these joint-play movements is a most important part of learning how to perform them correctly.

My course lasts twenty hours, and this is only just time enough
in which to demonstrate the normal movements of joint play at
every synovial joint in the body. No student after that can yet
consider himself trained in manipulative techniques — he has
only been exposed to them. He has yet to apply his examining
techniques to a painful joint. It is only then that he may hazard
a diagnosis of simple joint dysfunction and then pluck up courage

to perform a therapeutic manipulation. I have found that it takes about six months of preceptor training of an aware physician before he can expect to become a proficient user of manipulative techniques.

Manipulating joints is an art and, as with so many arts, not everyone can expect to be able to learn to use it. Perhaps there are two main reasons why joint manipulation has not found the wide acceptance that it merits in the practice of medicine; first, the user has not learned the proper techniques; and second, the user is simply inept at the art. It is so much easier to blame a modality of treatment for failure than it is to blame someone who perhaps never should be using the modality in the first place.

There is one pitfall in teaching and learning these techniques that must be stressed. The student must learn to elicit the normal joint-play movements of the limb, both on the right and left extremities. It is essential to be ambidextrous in this field.

I have tried to make it clear that joint manipulation is not the beginning and the end of the treatment of joint pain. This cannot be repeated too often. Therapeutic manipulation can only be expected to relieve the symptom of pain arising from joint dysfunction. Joint dysfunction impairs normal voluntary joint movement. Though the performance of normal voluntary joint movement depends on the integrity of the range of movement of joint play, there are obviously other factors which determine one's ability to have normal, painless joint movement and function. The muscles that act upon a joint, the ligaments that support the joint, the capsular structures of the joint, the hyaline cartilage of the joint, and the intra-articular fibrocartilages when present in the joint must also be anatomically normal and physiologically functional. Any pathological joint condition, whether simple joint dysfunction or some serious joint disease, affects to some extent all the anatomical structures that play a part in the functioning of the joint. All the affected structures need attention in treatment if a return to normalcy is to be expected. For instance, an atrophied muscle cannot be restored to normal if the joint that it moves is not free to move. Equally, normal joint movement is soon lost if the muscles that move it are weak or the ligaments that support it are damaged.

So, joint manipulation is one modality of treatment that may or may not have a place in the treatment of a painful joint. If it is not used when it is indicated, treatment will fail to alleviate the patient's symptoms; if it is used when it should not be, treatment will also fail to relieve the patient's symptoms and, indeed, may even make them worse.

To treat joint pain, it is necessary to be conversant with all available modalities of physical treatment. Intra-articular injections, the spraying or injecting of trigger points in muscles and ligaments, the judicious use of splints, supports, supporting bandages, and braces, and the proper use of rest may each prove to be the basis of successful treatment. Orthopedic surgery may hold the only hope for the relief of joint pain, but often this is only successful if the tenets of treatment which are advocated throughout this work are strictly adhered to.

When physical treatment is properly prescribed, it is likely to be useless if it is not properly applied. Casual technicians or office staff cannot be expected properly to administer any modality of physical treatment. I cannot advocate too strongly to my colleagues that they should use the services of properly trained and certified Registered Physical Therapists who are members in good standing of the American Physical Therapy Association.

There are too few Registered Physical Therapists to meet the needs of the public. There are too many untrained and unskilled technicians administering physical treatment without hindrance. It is important that students should be encouraged to become physical therapists, and that this profession should be made attractive.

In this book I have attempted to draw attention to one additional cause of joint pain — joint dysfunction — which can readily be treated by joint manipulation, a little-used modality of therapy. The hypothesis of joint play in no way vitiates the principles of the basic sciences of anatomy and physiology. The diagnosis of joint dysfunction in no way flouts the principles of the basic science of pathology.

My object in writing this book has been to bring joint manipulation into proper perspective for those who may have been previously biased against it as a form of "cultism." I hope that those who have not before used manipulative techniques may have found here an understanding of them and a way of correctly using them for the benefit of patients who are entitled to all the skills of treatment that are available.

Index

173

M7

FEB

DRAKE MEMORIAL LIBRARY
WITHDRAWN
THE COLLEGE AT BROCKPORT